101 CT Abdomen Solutions

101 CT Abdomen Solutions

Hariqbal Singh MD DMRD
Professor and Head
Department of Radiology
Shrimati Kashibai Navale Medical College
Pune, Maharashtra, India

Yasmeen Khan DMRE
Consultant
Department of Radiology
Shrimati Kashibai Navale Medical College
Pune, Maharashtra, India

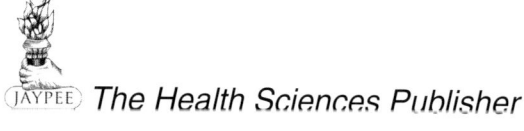

JAYPEE The Health Sciences Publisher
New Delhi | London | Philadelphia | Panama

Jaypee Brothers Medical Publishers (P) Ltd.

Headquarters
Jaypee Brothers Medical Publishers (P) Ltd.
4838/24, Ansari Road, Daryaganj
New Delhi 110 002, India
Phone: +91-11-43574357
Fax: +91-11-43574314
E-mail: jaypee@jaypeebrothers.com

Overseas Offices

J.P. Medical Ltd.
83, Victoria Street, London
SW1H 0HW (UK)
Phone: +44-20 3170 8910
Fax: +44(0)20 3008 6180
E-mail: info@jpmedpub.com

Jaypee Medical Inc.
325, Chestnut Street, Suite 412
Philadelphia, PA 19106, USA
Phone: +1 267-519-9789
E-mail: jpmed.us@gmail.com

Jaypee-Highlights Medical Publishers Inc.
City of Knowledge, Bld. 237, Clayton
Panama City, Panama
Phone: +1 507-301-0496
Fax: +1 507-301-0499
E-mail: cservice@jphmedical.com

Jaypee Brothers Medical Publishers (P) Ltd.
17/1-B, Babar Road, Block-B, Shaymali
Mohammadpur, Dhaka-1207
Bangladesh
Mobile: +08801912003485
E-mail: jaypeedhaka@gmail.com

Jaypee Brothers Medical Publishers (P) Ltd.
Bhotahity, Kathmandu, Nepal
Phone: +977-9741283608
E-mail: kathmandu@jaypeebrothers.com

Website: www.jaypeebrothers.com
Website: www.jaypeedigital.com

© 2016, Jaypee Brothers Medical Publishers

The views and opinions expressed in this book are solely those of the original contributor(s)/author(s) and do not necessarily represent those of editor(s) of the book.

All rights reserved. No part of this publication may be reproduced, stored or transmitted in any form or by any means, electronic, mechanical, photocopying, recording or otherwise, without the prior permission in writing of the publishers.

All brand names and product names used in this book are trade names, service marks, trademarks or registered trademarks of their respective owners. The publisher is not associated with any product or vendor mentioned in this book.

Medical knowledge and practice change constantly. This book is designed to provide accurate, authoritative information about the subject matter in question. However, readers are advised to check the most current information available on procedures included and check information from the manufacturer of each product to be administered, to verify the recommended dose, formula, method and duration of administration, adverse effects and contraindications. It is the responsibility of the practitioner to take all appropriate safety precautions. Neither the publisher nor the author(s)/editor(s) assume any liability for any injury and/or damage to persons or property arising from or related to use of material in this book.

This book is sold on the understanding that the publisher is not engaged in providing professional medical services. If such advice or services are required, the services of a competent medical professional should be sought.

Every effort has been made where necessary to contact holders of copyright to obtain permission to reproduce copyright material. If any have been inadvertently overlooked, the publisher will be pleased to make the necessary arrangements at the first opportunity.

Inquiries for bulk sales may be solicited at: jaypee@jaypeebrothers.com

101 CT Abdomen Solutions

First Edition: **2016**

ISBN: 978-93-5250-181-6

Printed at Sanat Printers

Dedicated to
*The unwearied, enduring, tolerant, and serene patients
who place themselves in the hands of
clinicians involved in research
in pursuit to alleviate their suffering
for restoration of health.*

*Radiology is a kindergarten
of logical rational coherent exploration and
balanced learning
and not dexterous adroit smugness
or learning egotism
cultivated by fake self-centeredness and egoism.*

—**Hariqbal Singh**

Preface

The huge response received following the publication of *101 Chest X-ray Solutions* and *101 MRI Brain Solutions*, prompted us to develop on *101 CT Abdomen Solutions*, which will hopefully be equally accepted by the readers. It provides a large bank of CT images on abdomen with cases seen in routine practice to more difficult cases of interest. With these images in mind, it will help the CT practitioner to interpret the possible diagnosis on abdominal CT during routine reporting practice. It will be an ideal reference for anyone involved with CT image interpretation. In many images, small arrow point is used to show the lesion. This is with an aim to provide better understanding for the reader. The importance of having a good knowledge of anatomy cannot be undermined and this has guided us to include a chapter on normal anatomy of Abdomen on CT imaging.

The book is meant for radiology residents, radiologists, general practitioners, other specialists, CT technical staff and those who have a special interest in CT imaging. It is meant for medical colleges and institutional libraries, departmental and CT standalone unit libraries.

The book is a compilation of cases developed by unified, consistent and cohesive endeavor of the panel of radiologists at Shrimati Kashibai Navale Medical College, Pune, Maharashtra, India.

Hariqbal Singh
Yasmeen Khan

Acknowledgments

We thank Professor MN Navale, Founder President, Sinhgad Technical Education Society and Dr AV Bhore, Dean, Shrimati Kashibai Navale Medical College, Pune, Maharashtra, India, for their kind acquiescence in this endeavor.

We are profusely extending our gratefulness to the consultants Varsha Rangankar, Santosh Konde, Abhijit Pawar, Amol Sasane, Aditi Dongre, Pooja Shah, Shripad Kamble, Patil Dharmendra, Varsha Sonawane, and Ajinkya Kolse for their genuine help in building up this educational entity.

We are profusely gratified to the radiology residents Swati Shah, Vikram Shende, Jarvis Pereira, Priya Bhole, Prasad Patil, Punit Agrawal, Swapnil Raut, Amar Sangapwad and Prajakta Jagtap for their genuine help in correction of the manuscript.

Our gratitude to Anna Bansode and Sachin Babar for their clerical help.

We are thankful and grateful to the God Almighty and mankind who have allowed us to have this wonderful experience.

Contents

CT Anatomy: Abdomen and Pelvis — 1

SECTION 1 Esophagus

1. Hiatus Hernia — 19
2. Esophageal Carcinoma — 21
3. Leiomyomatosis of Esophagus — 23

SECTION 2 Diaphragm

4. Eventration — 27
5. Eventration of Diaphragm with Duplication of Inferior Vena Cava — 29

SECTION 3 Stomach

6. Gastrointestinal Stromal Tumor — 33
7. Gastric Malignanacy — 35

SECTION 4 Duodenum

8. Carcinoma Duodenum — 41

SECTION 5 Small Bowel

9. Small Bowel Obstruction — 45
10. Ileocecal Lymphoma — 47
11. Small Bowel Gastrointestinal Stromal Tumor — 49
12. Angiodysplasia of Jejunum — 51
13. Ileal Carcinoma — 53
14. Pneumatosis Intestinalis — 55
15. Midgut Volvulus — 57

SECTION 6 Appendix

16. Acute Appendicitis — 61
17. Appendicular Abscess — 63

SECTION 7 Colon

18. Intussusception — 67
19. Nontoxic Megacolon — 70

20.	Sigmoid Diverticulitis	72
21.	Abdominal Koch's	74
22.	Carcinoma Sigmoid	77

SECTION 8 Rectum

23.	Carcinoma Rectum	81

SECTION 9 Liver

24.	Focal Fatty Liver	87
25.	Simple Hepatic Cyst	89
26.	Budd-Chiari Syndrome	91
27.	Liver Laceration	94
28.	Hepatic Abscess	97
29.	Hepatic Hydatid Cyst	100
30.	Hepatic Hemangioma	103
31.	Focal Nodular Hyperplasia	106
32.	Hepatic Adenoma	108
33.	Hepatic Angiomyolipoma	110
34.	Hepatocellular Carcinoma	112
35.	Hepatic Metastases	115
36.	Hepatoblastoma	118
37.	Intrahepatic Cholangiocarcinoma	120
38.	Extrahepatic Cholangiocarcinoma	123
39.	Transient Hepatic Attenuation Difference	125

SECTION 10 Gallbladder

40.	Choledochal Cyst	129
41.	Acalculus Cholecystitis	131
42.	Acute Calculus Cholecystitis	133
43.	Emphysematous Cholecystitis	136
44.	Choledocholithiasis	138
45.	Porcelain Gallbladder	140
46.	Carcinoma Gallbladder	142

SECTION 11 Pancreas

47.	Acute Pancreatitis	147
48.	Pancreatic Pseudocyst	149
49.	Necrotizing Pancreatitis	153
50.	Periampullary Carcinoma with Metastases	155

SECTION 12 Spleen

51.	Splenunculus	161
52.	Splenic Trauma	163
53.	Splenic Abscess	166

SECTION 13 Vascular

54. Superior Mesenteric Artery Syndrome	171
55. Superior Mesenteric Artery Thrombosis	173
56. Accessory Renal Artery Stenosis	176
57. Aneurysm of Abdominal Aorta	178
58. Inferior Vena Cava Thrombus	180
59. Aortic Thrombus	182
60. Portal Vein Thrombosis	184

SECTION 14 Adrenal

61. Adrenal Adenoma	189
62. Pheochromocytoma	192
63. Adrenal Metastases	194

SECTION 15 Renal

64. Renal Aplasia	199
65. Dysplastic Kidney	201
66. Polycystic Kidneys	203
67. Pelviureteric Junction Obstruction	205
68. Obstructive Uropathy	208
69. Emphysematous Pyelonephritis	215
70. Renal Vein Thrombosis	217
71. Renal Laceration	219
72. Renal Angiomyolipoma	221
73. Wilms' Tumor	223
74. Renal Cell Carcinoma	226

SECTION 16 Urinary Bladder

75. Vesical Calculus	231
76. Urinary Bladder Diverticulum	233
77. Cystitis	235
78. Carcinoma Urinary Bladder	237

SECTION 17 Prostate

79. Carcinoma Prostate	243

SECTION 18 Scrotum

80. Hydrocele	247
81. Testicular Trauma	249
82. Seminoma	251
83. Undescended Testis	253

SECTION 19 Penis

84. Penile Carcinoma	257

SECTION 20 Uterus

85. Broad Ligament Fibroid	261
86. Hydrometrocolpos	263
87. Pyometra	265
88. Endometrial Carcinoma	267
89. Carcinoma Cervix	270
90. Vaginal Carcinoma	272
91. Ureterovaginal Fistula	274
92. Vulval Carcinoma	276

SECTION 21 Ovary

93. Ovarian Vein Thrombosis	281
94. Ovarian Tumor	283

SECTION 22 Abdominal Wall

95. Abdominal Wall Sarcoma	289
96. Abdominal Wall Hernia	291

SECTION 23 Miscellaneous

97. Inguinal Hernia	297
98. Omental Infarction	300
99. Primitive Neuroectodermal Tumor	302
100. Fetus-in-Fetu	304
101. Lymphangioma	306

Index 309

Introduction

PHYSICAL PRINCIPLE OF CT SCAN IMAGING

CT was invented in 1972 by British engineer, Sir Godfrey Newbold Hounsfield in Hayes, United Kingdom at EMI Central Research Laboratories using X-rays. EMI laboratories is best known today for its music and recording business. About the same time South Africa-born American physicist, Allan McLeod Cormack of Tufts University in Massachusetts independently invented a similar process, and both shared the 1979 Nobel Prize.

The first clinical CT scan was installed in 1974. The initial systems were dedicated only to head scanning due to small gantry, but soon this was overcome and whole body CT system with larger gantry, became available in 1976.

Basic principle is to obtain a tomogram having thickness in millimeters of the region of interest using pencil beam X-radiation. The radiation transmitted through the patient is counted by scintillation detector. This information when fed in the computer is analyzed by mathematical algorithms and reconstructed as a tomographic image by the computer so as to provide an insight into the structure being studied (Table 1).

Developments in CT Technology

Conventional Axial CT (Table 1)

Table 1: Generations of CT scan

Generation of CT scan	Motion of X-ray tube-detector system	Stationary detectors	X-ray beam type
First	Translate-Rotate	Two detectors	Pencil beam
Second	Translate-Rotate	Multiple detectors up to 30	Narrow fan beam (10°)
Third	Rotate-Rotate	Multiple detectors up to 750	Wide fan beam (50°)
Fourth	Rotate-Fixed	Ring of 1500–4500 detectors	Fan beam
Fifth	Rotate-Fixed	Two rings of 1500–4500 detectors with two tubes	Fan beam

Spiral/Helical CT

Spiral CT uses the conventional technology in conjunction with slip ring technology, which simultaneously provides high voltage for X-ray tube, low voltage for control unit and transmits digital data from detector array. Slip ring is a circular instrument with sliding bushes that enables the gantry to rotate continuously while the patient table moves into the gantry simultaneously, thus three-dimensional volume rendered image can be obtained. The advantages over the conventional scanner are the reduced scan time, reduced radiation exposure and reduced contrast requirement with superior information.

Electron Beam CT (EBCT)

In EBCT, both the X-ray source and the detectors are stationary. High energy focused electron beam is magnetically steered on the tungsten target to emit X-rays, which pass through the subject on to the detectors and image is acquired. EBCT is particularly used for faster imaging in cardiac studies.

Multislice/Multidetector CT (MDCT)

Spiral CT uses single row of detectors, resulting in a single slice per gantry rotation. Multislice CT, multiple detector arrays are used resulting in multiple slices per gantry rotation. In addition, fan beam geometry of spiral CT is replaced by cone beam geometry.

The major advantages over spiral CT are improved spatial and temporal resolution, reduced image noise, faster and longer anatomic coverage, and increased concentration of intravenous contrast.

Dual Source CT

The dual energy technology of the new Flash CT provides higher contrast between normal and abnormal tissues making it easier to see abnormalities while reducing radiation. With its two rotating X-ray tubes, enhanced speed and power allows children to be screened more effectively. It turns off the radiation when it comes close to sensitive tissue areas of the body like thyroid, breasts, or eye lens.

Pediatric patients benefit because they do not need to hold breath or lay completely still during the examination and they do not have to be sedated.

Hounsfield Units

CT numbers recognized by the computer are from (–) 1000 to (+) 1000, i.e. a range of 2000 Hounsfield units which are present in the image as 2000 shades of gray, but our eye cannot precisely discriminate between these 2000 different shades.

Hounsfield scale assigns attenuation value of water as zero (HU 0), and other tissues their attenuation value as compared to water as given in Table 2.

Table 2: Attenuation value of various tissues on CT scan

Tissue	Attenuation value in HU
Air	(–)1000
Lung	(–) 400 to (–) 800
Fat	(–) 40 to (–) 100
Water	0
Fresh blood	55 to 65
Soft tissue	40 to 80
Bone	400 to 1000

Window Level (WL) and Window Width (WW)

To permit the viewer to understand the image, only a restricted number of HU are put on view and this is accomplished by setting the WL and WW on the console to a suitable range of Hounsfield units, depending on the tissue, for interpreting the image. The expression WL represents the central Hounsfield value of all the Hounsfield numbers within the WW. Tissues with CT numbers outside this array are shown as either black or white. Both the WL and WW can be set on the displayed image as desired by the viewer. On CT examination of the chest, a WW of 300 to 350 and WL of 35 to 45 are chosen to image the mediastinum (soft tissue window) whereas WW of 1500 and WL of 0 is used to assess the lung.

Image Reconstruction

The acquisition of volumetric data using spiral CT means that the images can be postprocessed in ways appropriate to the clinical situation.

Multiplanar reformatting (MPR) is by taking standard axial images and subject to the three-dimensional array of CT numbers obtained with a series of contiguous slices; and can be viewed in sagittal, coronal, oblique and paraxial planes (Figs 1A to C).

Three-Dimensional Imaging

Many fractures like fracture of the mandible associated with frontal bone with or without walls of sinuses can be reconstructed into a 3-dimensional image (Figs 2A to D).

CT Angiography

CT angiography (CTA) sequence is created subsequent to intravenous contrast, images are acquired in the arterial phase and then reconstructed and exhibited in 2D or 3D format. This performance is used for imaging the aorta, renal, cerebral, coronary and peripheral arteries (Figs 3 to 5).

CT is readily available in most hospitals and stand-alone CT centers. It is fast imaging modality and provides with cross-sectional high-resolution images. Data acquired on axial scans can be used for multiplanar and 3D reconstructions.

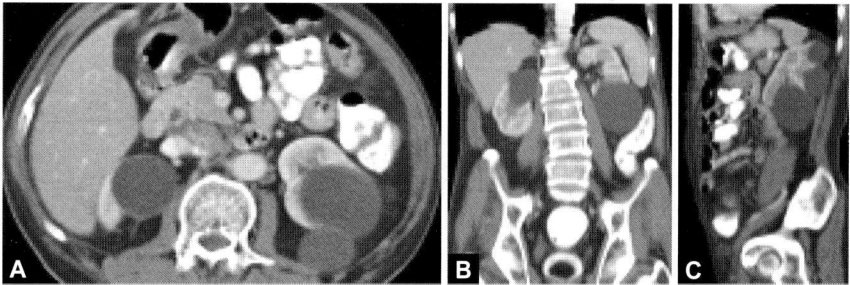

Figs 1A to C Bilateral renal cysts seen in axial section (A) are reformatted into sagittal; (B) and coronal; (C) planes

xviii 101 CT Abdomen Solutions

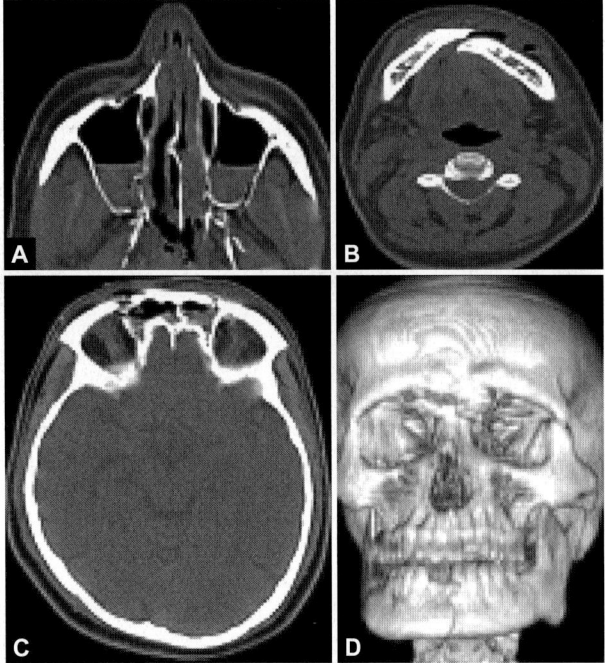

Figs 2A to D Fracture of body of mandible and frontal bone with bilateral maxillary hemosinus. D shows the 3D image of face including mandible

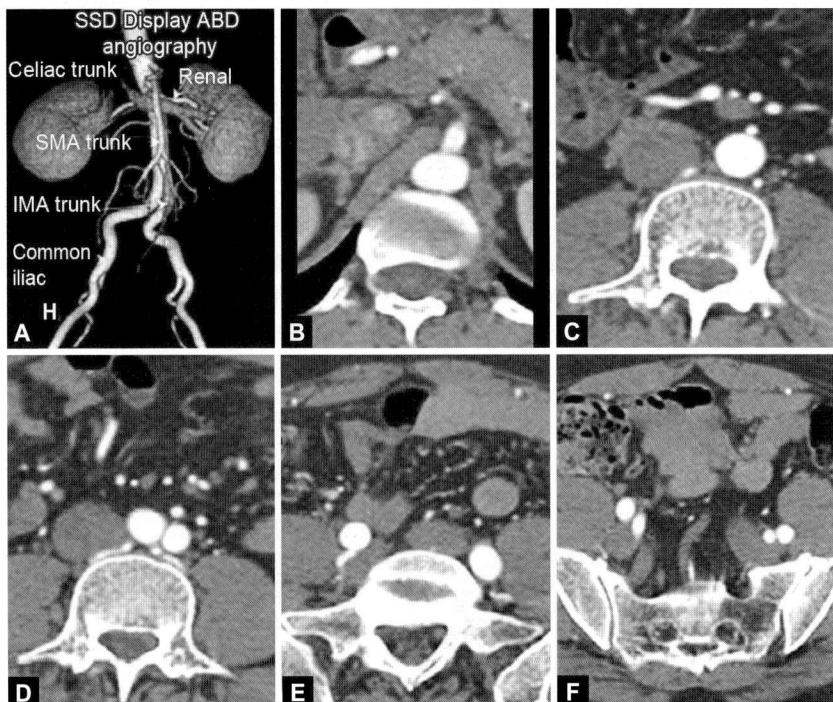

Figs 3A to F CT abdominal angiography

Introduction **xix**

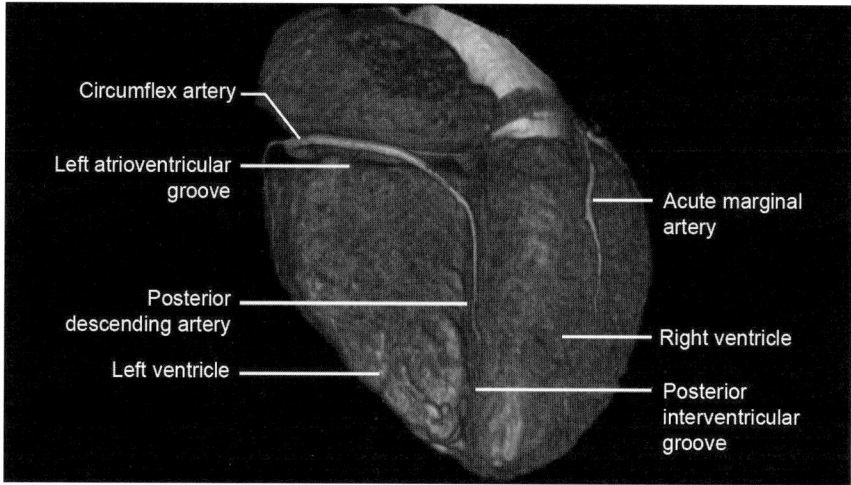

Fig. 4 Volume rendered image—posterior coronal plane shows coronary arteries *(For color version, see plate 1)*

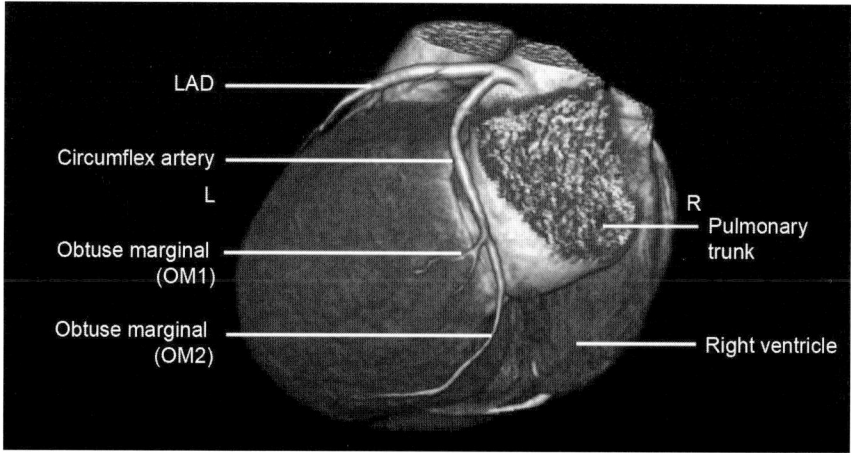

Fig. 5 Volume rendered image—posterior oblique coronal plane shows coronary arteries *(For color version, see plate 1)*

It detects subtle differences between body tissues. However, it uses X-rays which have radiation hazards, CT need contrast media for enhanced soft tissue contrast. Contrast is contraindicated in asthma, cardiac disease, renal and certain thyroid conditions.

Plate 1

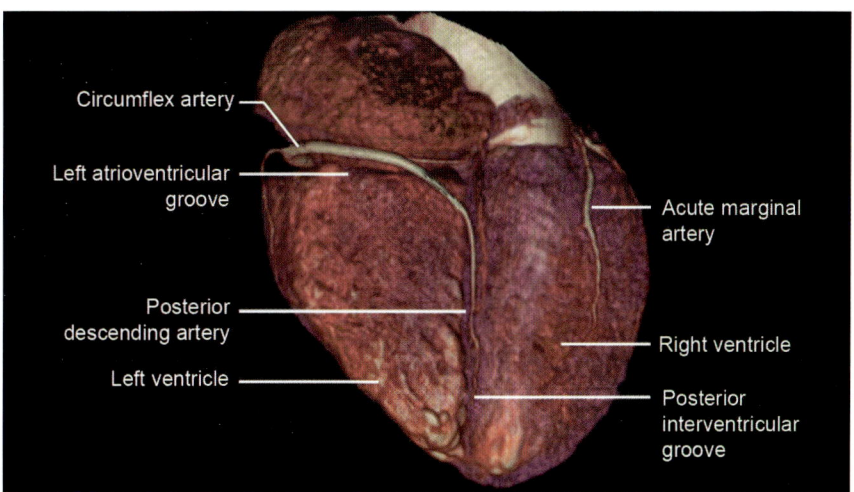

Fig. 4 Volume rendered image posterior coronal plane shows coronary arteries (Introduction)

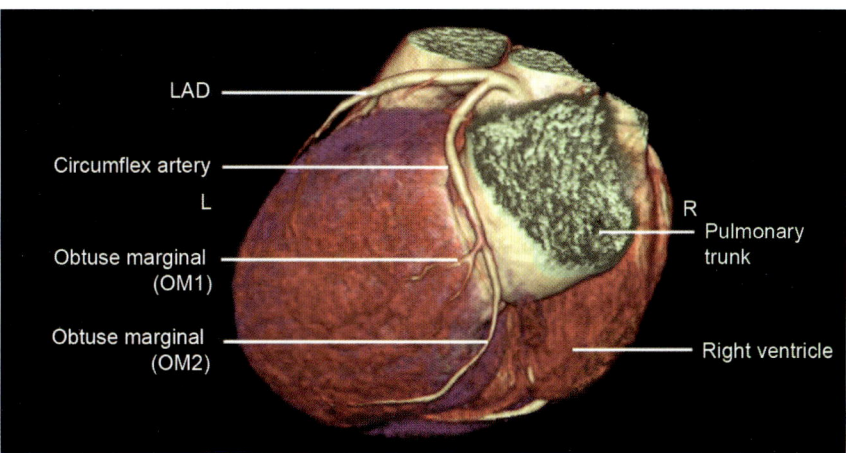

Fig. 5 Volume rendered image posterior oblique coronal plane shows coronary arteries (Introduction)

Plate 2

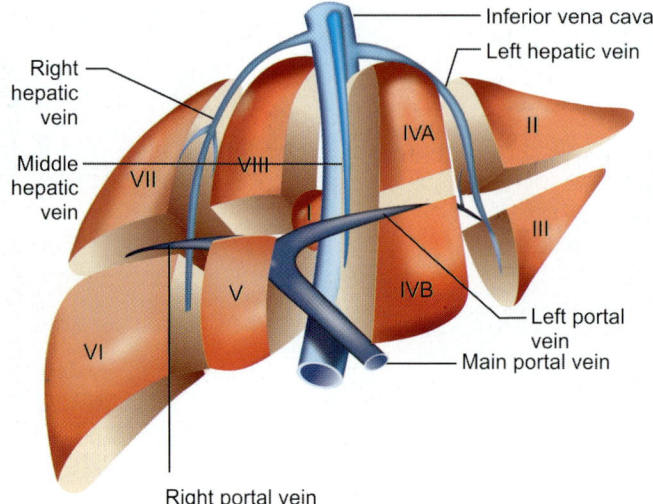

Fig. 1 Anatomy of liver segments (CT Anatomy: Abdomen and Pelvis)

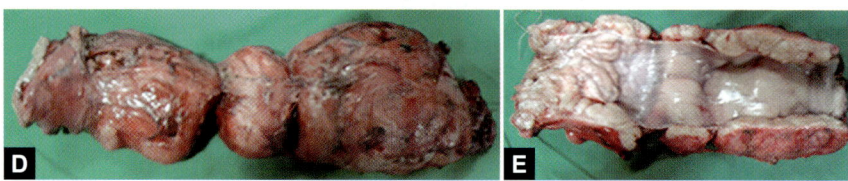

Figs 1D and E (Case 3)

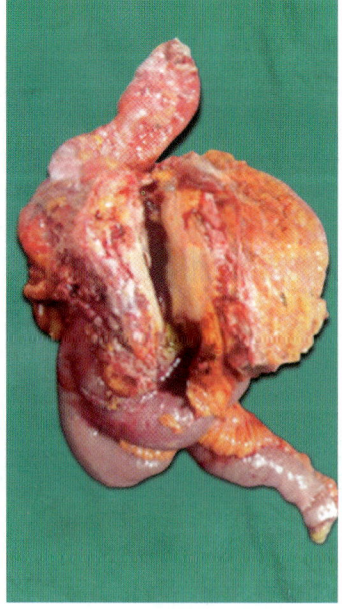

Fig. 1C (Case 10)

Plate 3

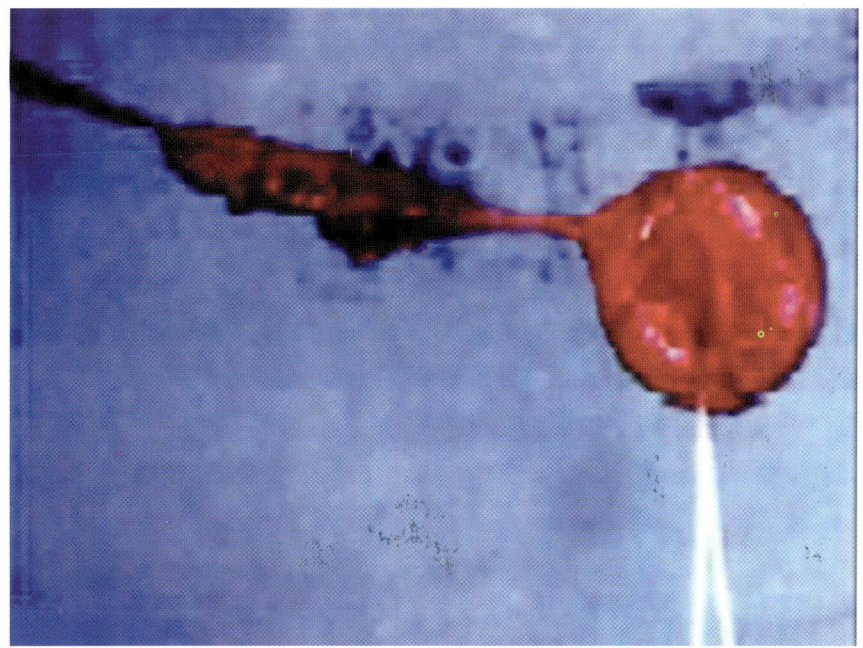

Fig. 1E (Case 40)

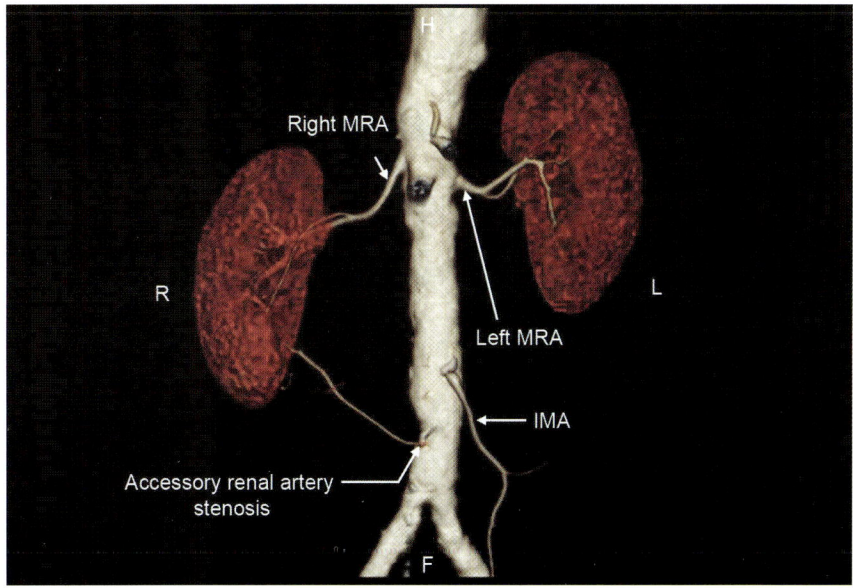

Fig. 1 (Case 56)

Plate 4

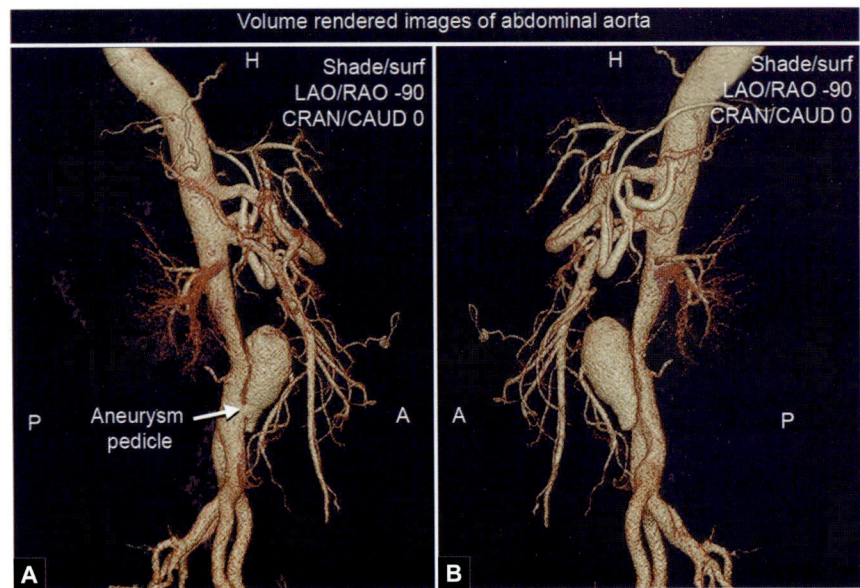

Figs 1A and B (Case 57)

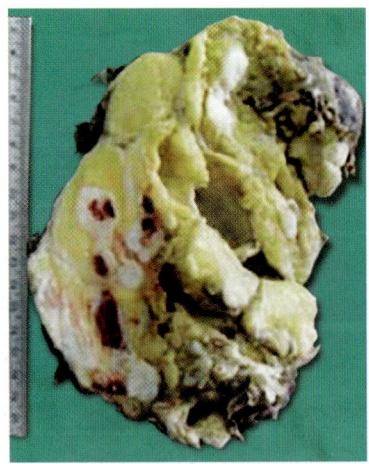

Fig. 1D (Case 100)

CT Anatomy: Abdomen and Pelvis

LIVER

Functional segmental anatomy of liver is based on distribution of three hepatic veins. Middle hepatic vein divides the liver into right and left lobes. Left hepatic vein divides the left lobe into medial and lateral parts. Right hepatic vein divides the right lobe into the anterior and posterior parts. An imaginary transverse line through the right and left portal vein divides these parts into anterior and posterior segments which are numbered counterclockwise from the inferior vena cava.

The Couinaud classification of liver anatomy divides the liver into eight functionally indepedent segments. Each segment has its own vascular inflow, outflow and biliary drainage. In the center of each segment there is a branch of the portal vein, hepatic artery and bile duct. The numbering of the segments is in a clockwise manner (Figs 1 and 2A to F).

Segment 1 (caudate lobe) is located posteriorly and extends between fissure of the ligamentum venosum anteriorly and the inferior vena cava posteriorly.

The longitudinal plane of the right hepatic vein divides segment 8 from segment 7 in the superior portion of the liver and in the inferior portion of the liver segment 5 from segment 6.

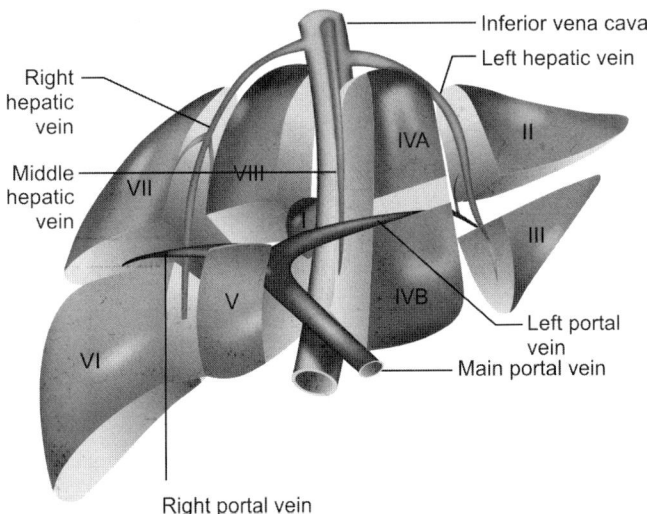

Fig. 1 Anatomy of liver segments *(For color version see Plate 2)*

2 101 CT Abdomen Solutions

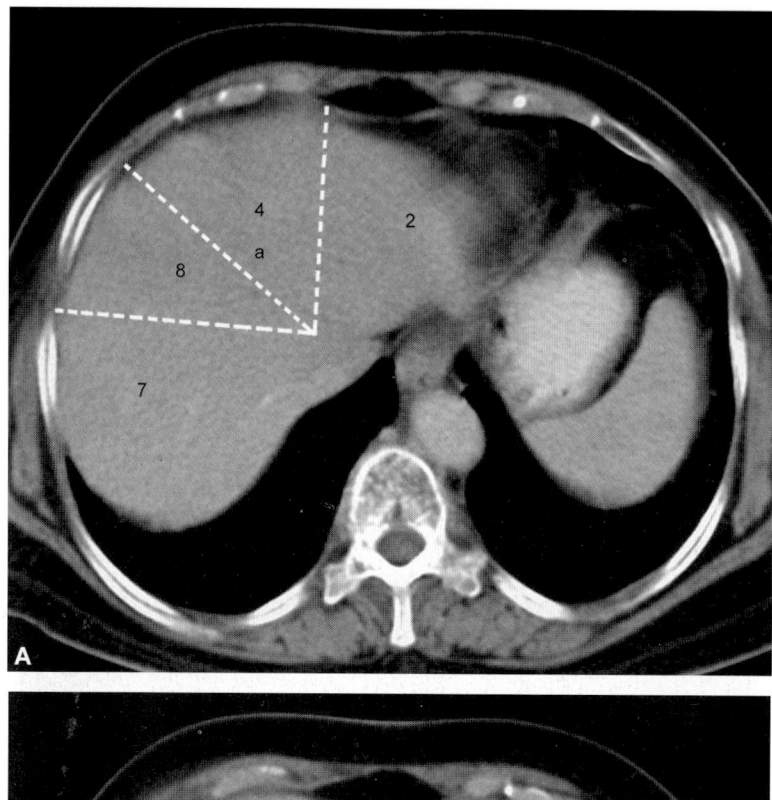

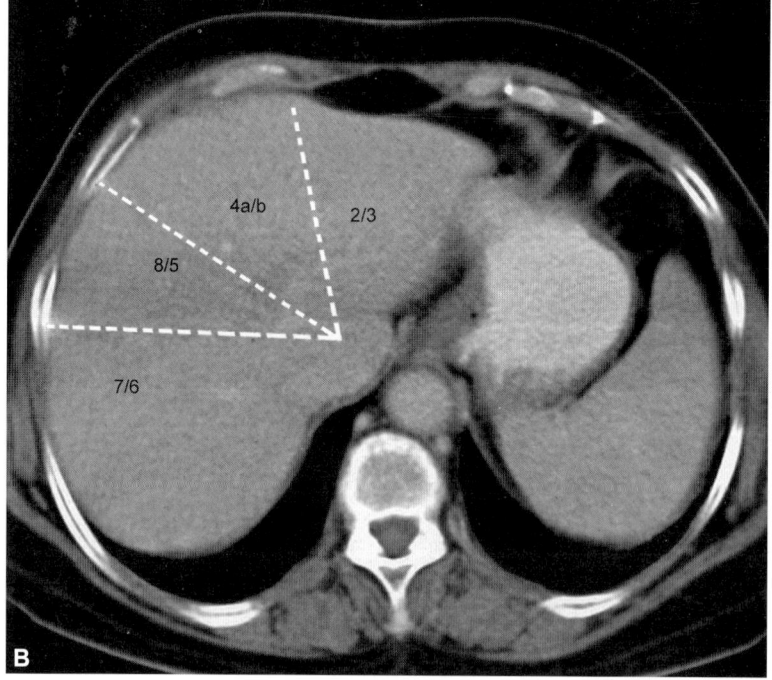

Figs 2A and B

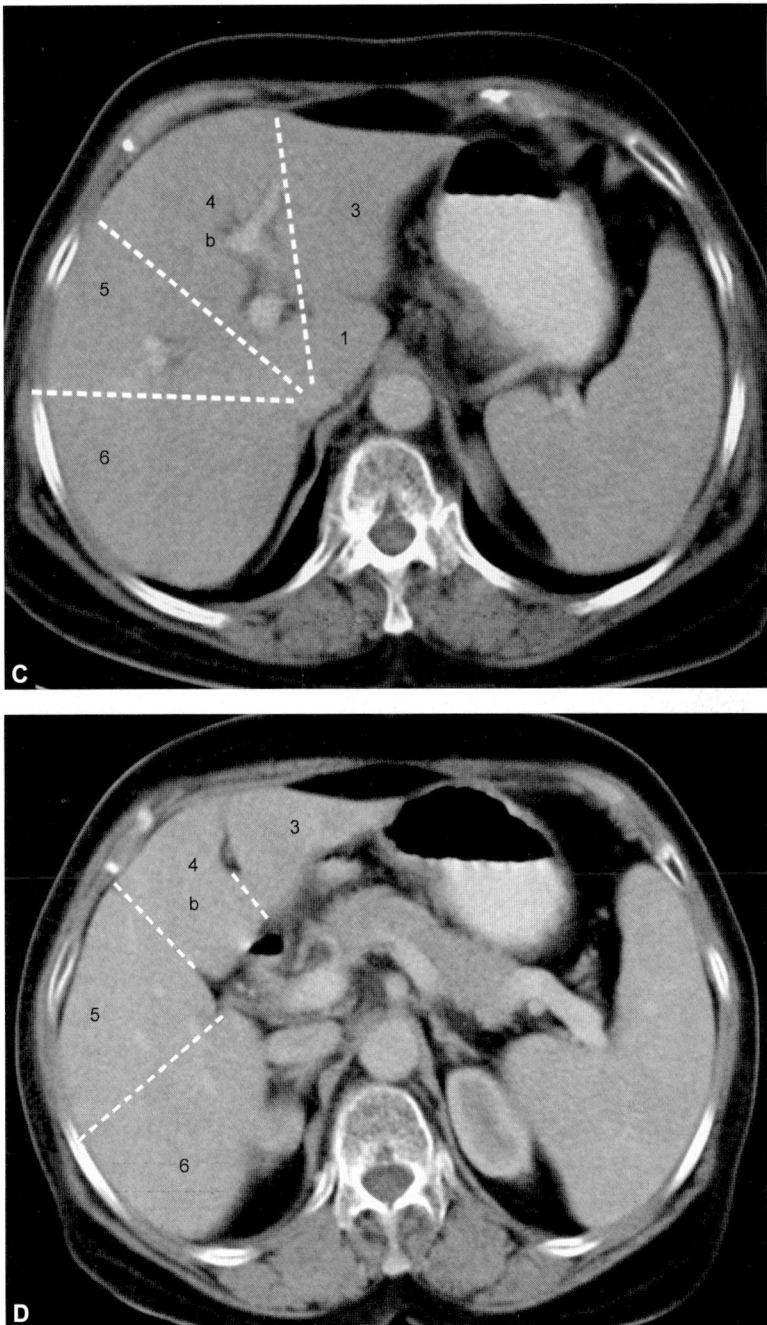

Figs 2C and D

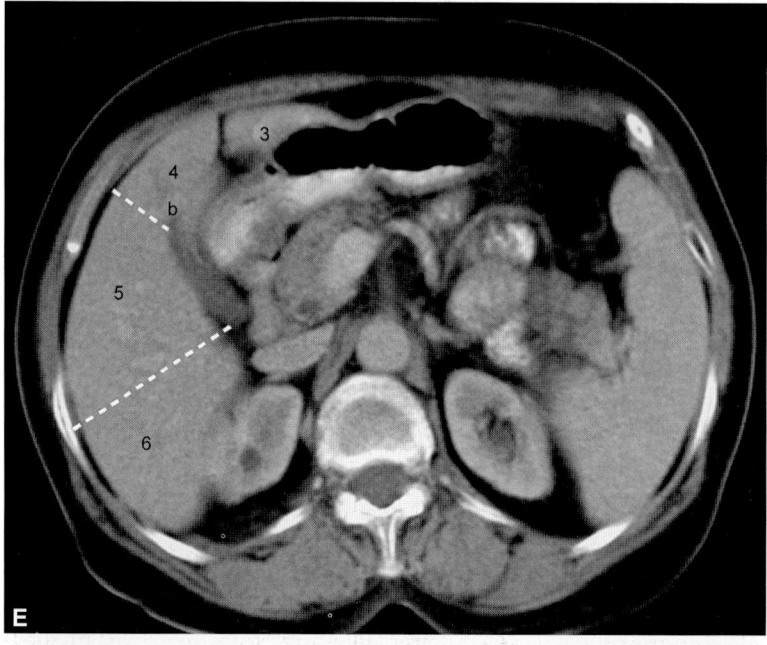

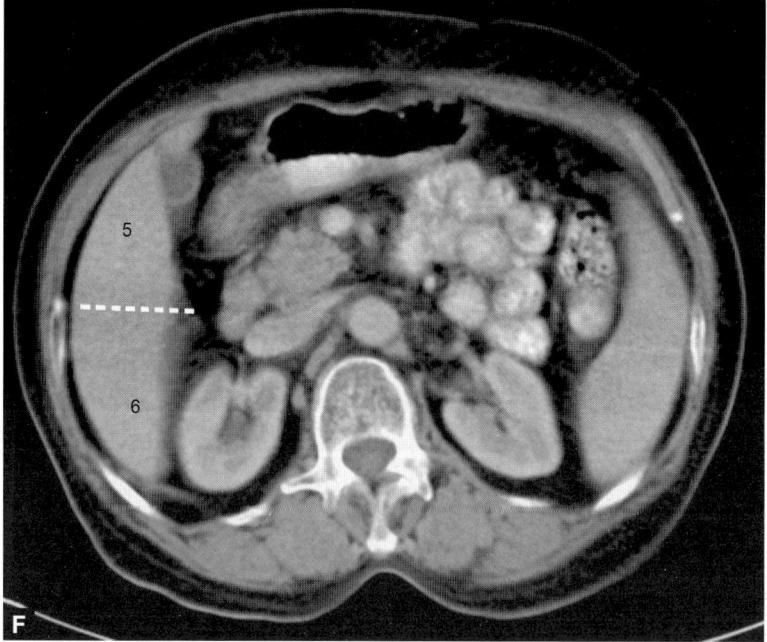

Figs 2E and F

The longitudinal plane of the middle hepatic vein through the gallbladder fossa separates segment 4a from segment 8 in the superior liver and segment 4b from segment 5 in the inferior liver.

The longitudinal plane of the left hepatic vein and fissure of the ligamentum teres separates segment 4a from segment 2 in the superior liver and segment 4b from segment 3 in the inferior liver.

The axial plane of the left portal vein separates segment 4a superiorly from segment 4b inferiorly and segment 2 superiorly from segment 3 inferiorly in the left lobe.

The axial plane of the right portal vein separates segment 8 and segment 7 superiorly from segment 5 and segment 6 inferiorly in the right lobe.

Normal liver has a precontrast attenuation value of 45-65 HU and maximum enhancement occurs at 50-60 seconds after administration of contrast. Normal liver has a size up to 13 centimeters. Normal portal vein is 10-13 mm in diameter (Figs 2G to N).

GALLBLADDER

Normal gallbladder is up to 10 cm long and 4 cm wide. It has a normal wall thickness up to 3 mm. Gallbladder may have septae (Figs 2M and N). Bifid appearance is due to longitudinal septum. Phrygian cap gallbladder is due to kink or septum at the neck. Ectopic gallbladder can be seen beneath the left lobe of liver or even in retro hepatic location. Floating gallbladder can result from loose peritoneal attachments.

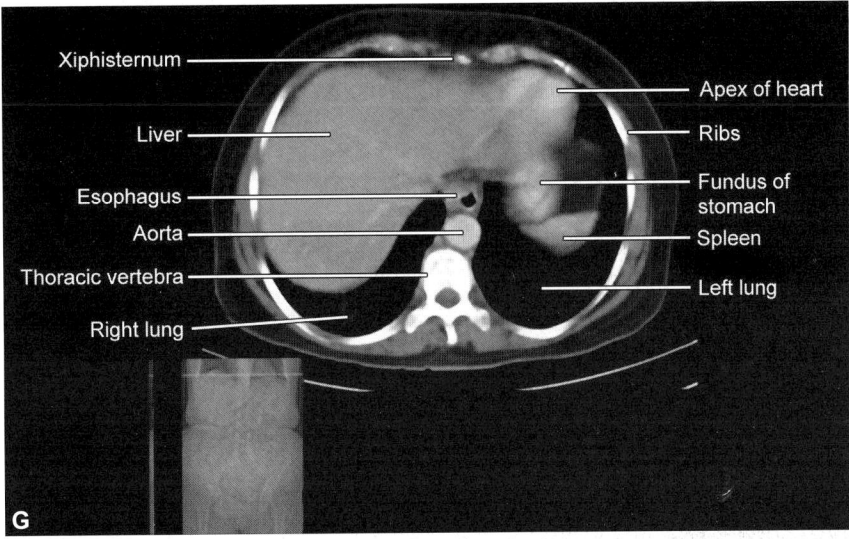

Fig. 2G

6 101 CT Abdomen Solutions

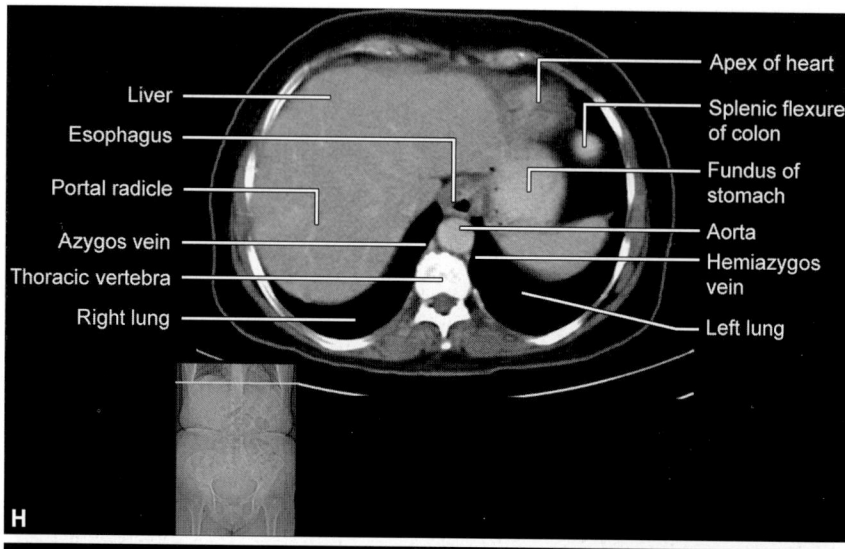

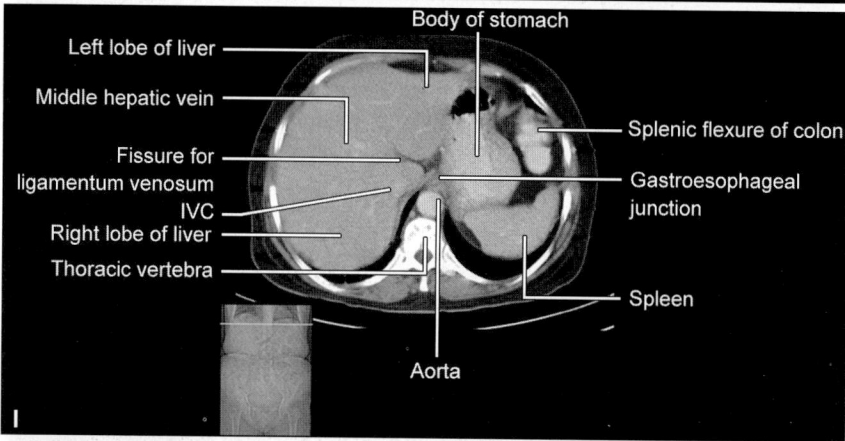

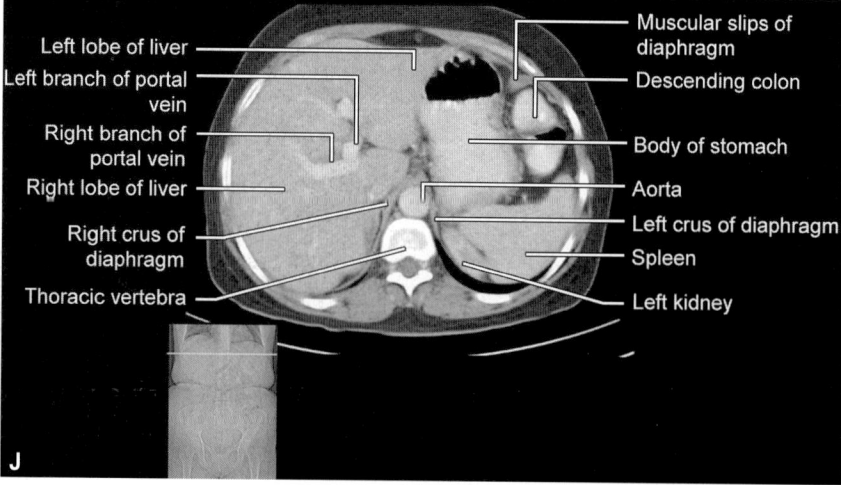

Figs 2H to J

CT Anatomy: Abdomen and Pelvis

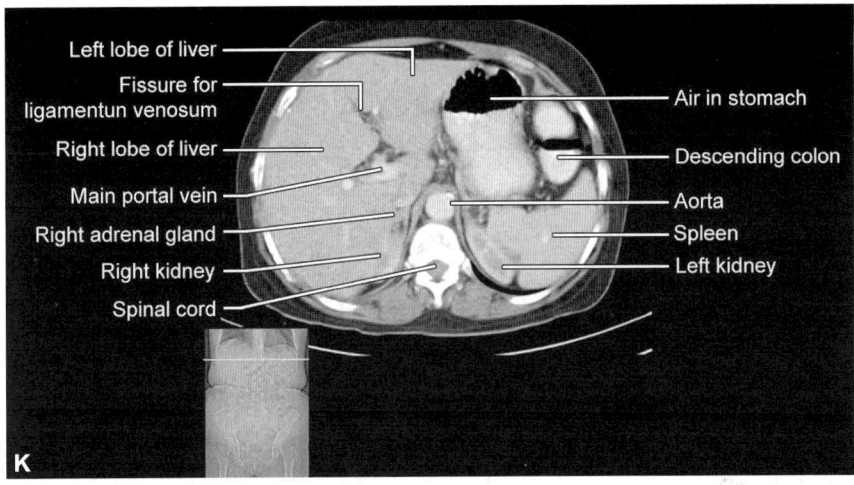

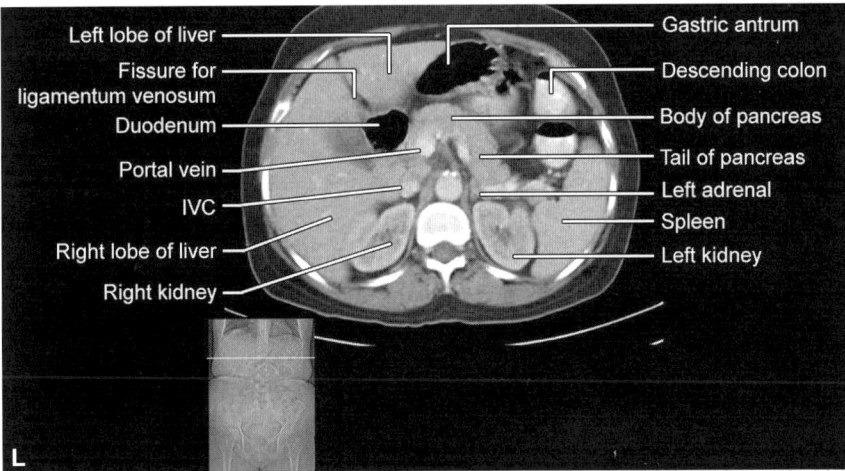

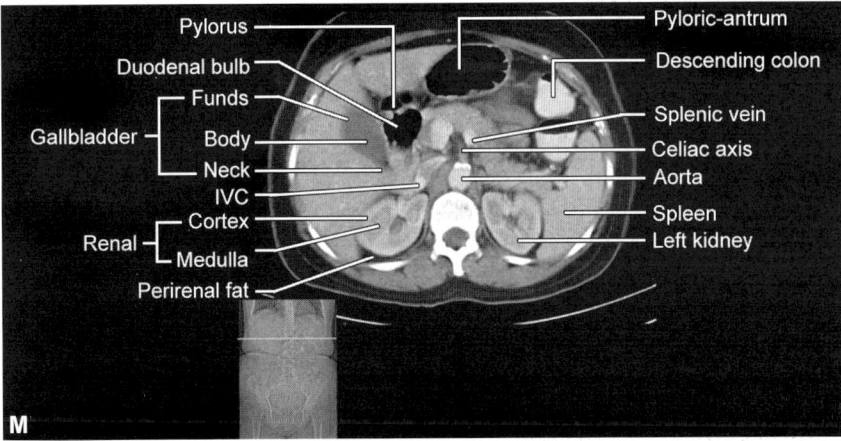

Figs 2K to M

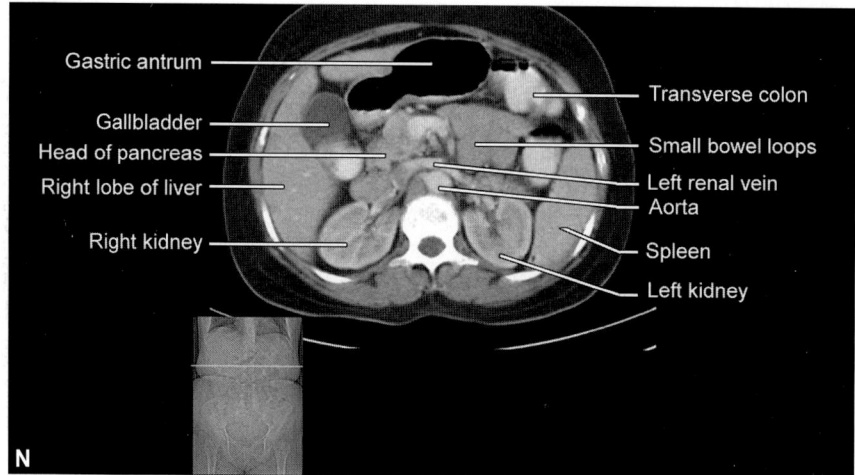

Fig. 2N

Normal cystic duct is 2 cm long and 2 mm wide. Maximum diameter of normal common bile duct in an adult is 2–5 mm. Post cholecystectomy it can be up to 7 mm. Normal width increases by 1mm per decade in elderly over 60 years of age.

PANCREAS

It develops during the fourth week of gestation as the second endodermal diverticulum from foregut. The dorsal diverticulum forms the dorsal pancreas. Ventral diverticulum forms the ventral pancreas as well as the liver, gallbladder and bile ducts.

The main pancreatic duct is known as the duct of Wirsung. The angle between the pancreatic duct and common bile duct at their joining point is between 5° and 30°. These ducts open into second part of duodenum through the ampulla of Vater which has a sphincter called the sphincter of Oddi.

The entire length of pancreas is 10–15 cm. Pancreatic tail is up to 1.6 cm thick; body is up to 1.1 cm thick and the head ranges from 1–2 cm in thickness (Figs 2L to O).

Annular pancreas is a congenital anomaly in which the duodenum is enclosed on all sides by pancreas as a result of abnormal migration of ventral pancreas.

SPLEEN

Spleen is formed during fifth week of gestational age from mesenchymal cells between layers of dorsal mesogastrium. Accessory spleen can be seen in 10–30% of patients. Spleen can even be attached to left testis or ovary as there is a close relationship between the left gonadal anlage and the splenic precursor mesenchymal cells (Splenogonadal fusion). It has a weight up to 200 g and a length of 11 cm. The CT value of spleen is 5 HU less than the liver.

GASTROINTESTINAL SYSTEM

The gastrointestinal system originates from a pouch like extension of yolk sac starting from 6 weeks of gestational age. The foregut is supplied by celiac artery, midgut by superior mesenteric artery and the hindgut by inferior mesenteric artery.

Upper gastrointestinal system starts from mouth and continues into oropharynx which continues into esophagus. Esophagus is a 25 cm long tubular structure which opens into the stomach via gastro esophageal junction. Parts of stomach are the fundus, body, greater and lesser curvatures, antrum and pylorus. Walls are 3–5 mm thick except in pylorus where it can be up to 7 mm thick (Figs 2H to O).

Small intestine can be up to 6 m long and extends from pyloric orifice of stomach up to ileocaecal valve. Duodenum is one feet long, jejunum is around 10 feet and ileum is upto 8 feet (Figs 2N to T). Fifteen centimeters long mesentery is located between ileocaecal junction and ligament of Treitz. Circular folds of small bowel are called as valvulae conniventes.

Rule of three for normal small bowel states that its walls are 3 mm thick, valvulae conniventes are 3 mm thick, there are less than 3 air fluid levels and the diameter is up to 3 cm.

Large intestine is 1.5 m long and extends from ileum to anus. Its parts are caecum, ascending colon, hepatic flexure of colon, transverse colon, splenic flexure, descending colon, sigmoid colon, rectum and anal canal (Figs 2O to T, 3A to C, 3E and 4).

Peritoneal spaces above transverse colon are:
- Spaces on the right
  - Right subphrenic space
  - Anterior and posterior right subhepatic space

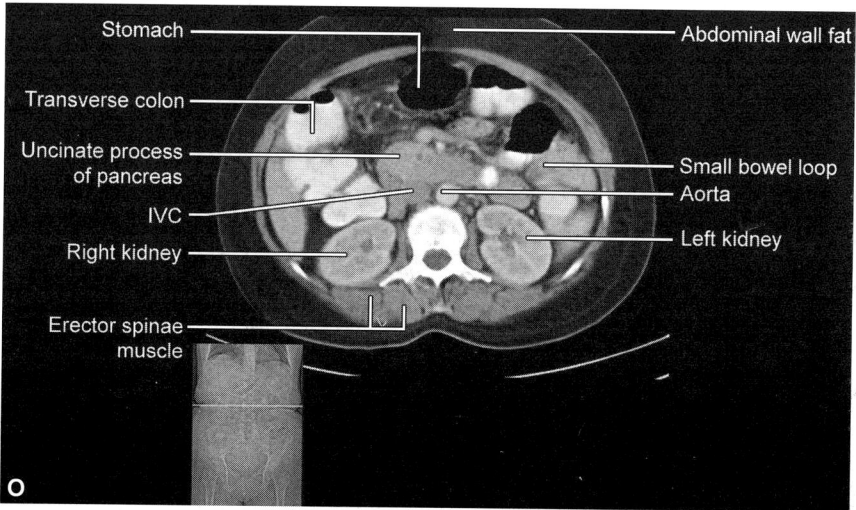

Fig. 2O

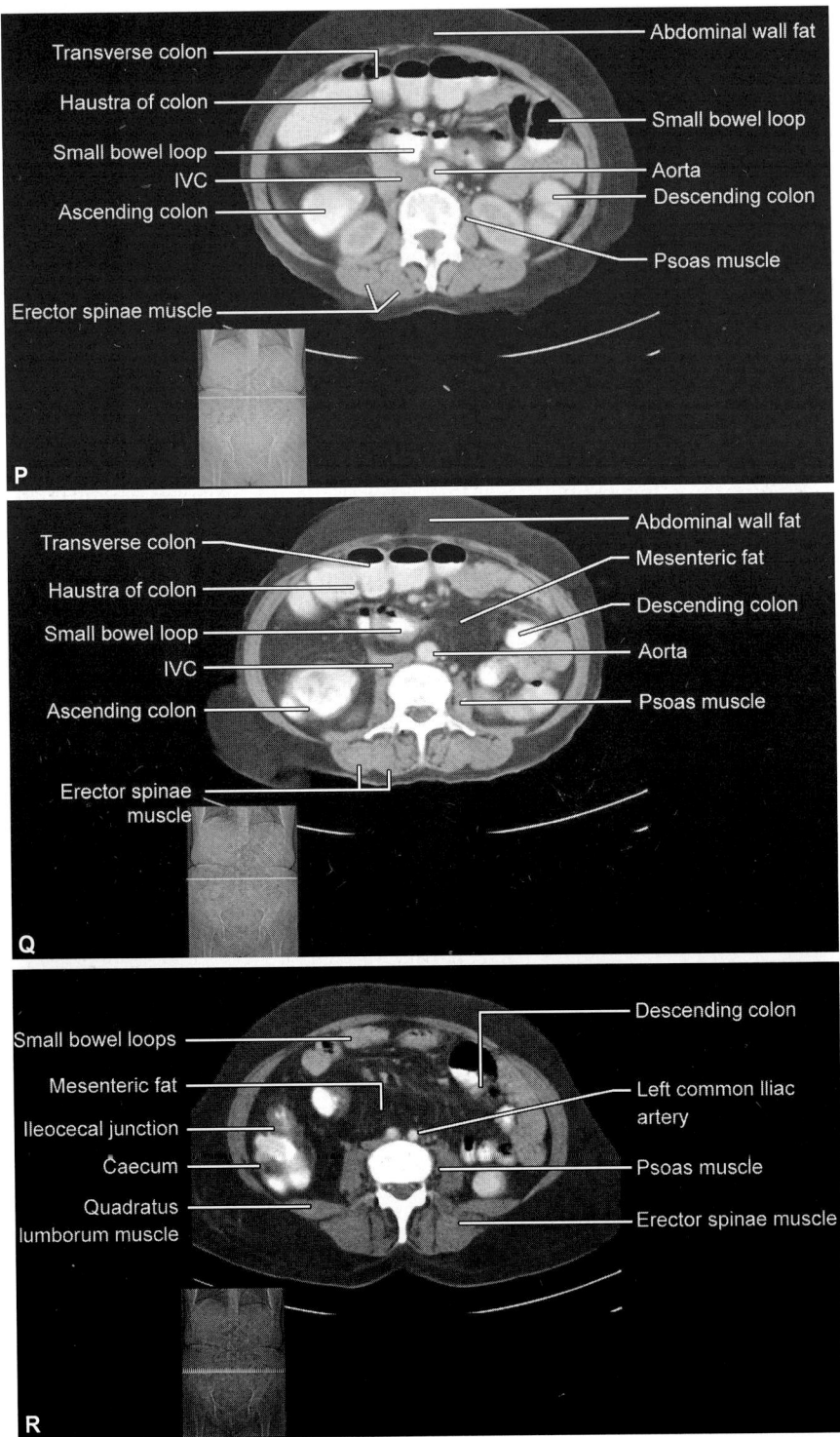

Figs 2P to R

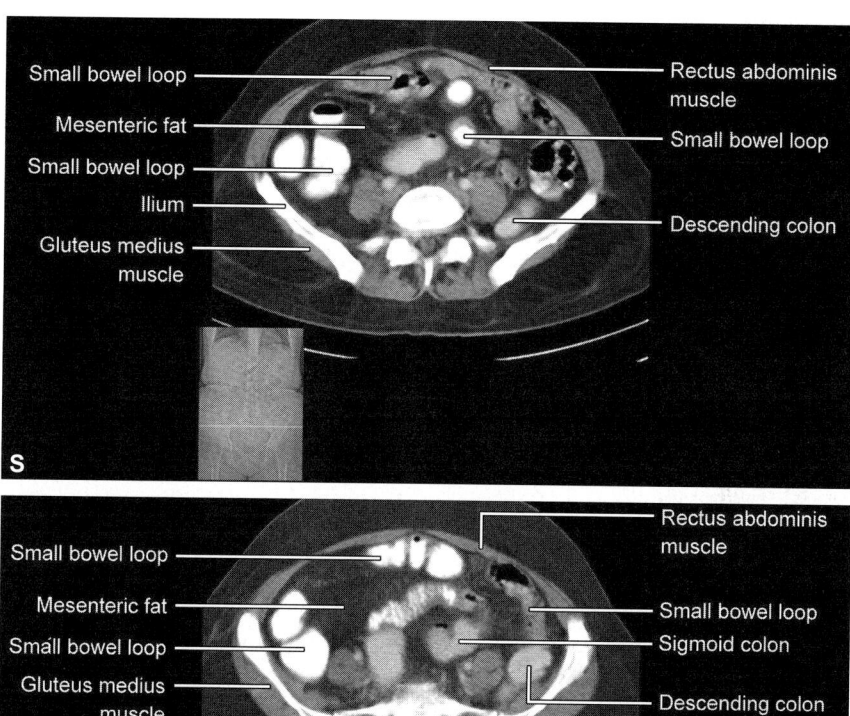

Figs 2S and T

Figs 2A to T Axial CT sections of abdomen

- Bare area of liver
- Lesser sac
- Spaces on the left
  - Left subphrenic space
  - Left subhepatic space
  - Perisplenic space

Peritoneal spaces below transverse colon are:
- Superior and Inferior Ileocecal recesses
- Retrocecal space
- Right and left paracolic gutters
- Intersigmoid recess.

Two folds of peritoneum supporting a structure within the peritoneal cavity together form a structure known as ligament.

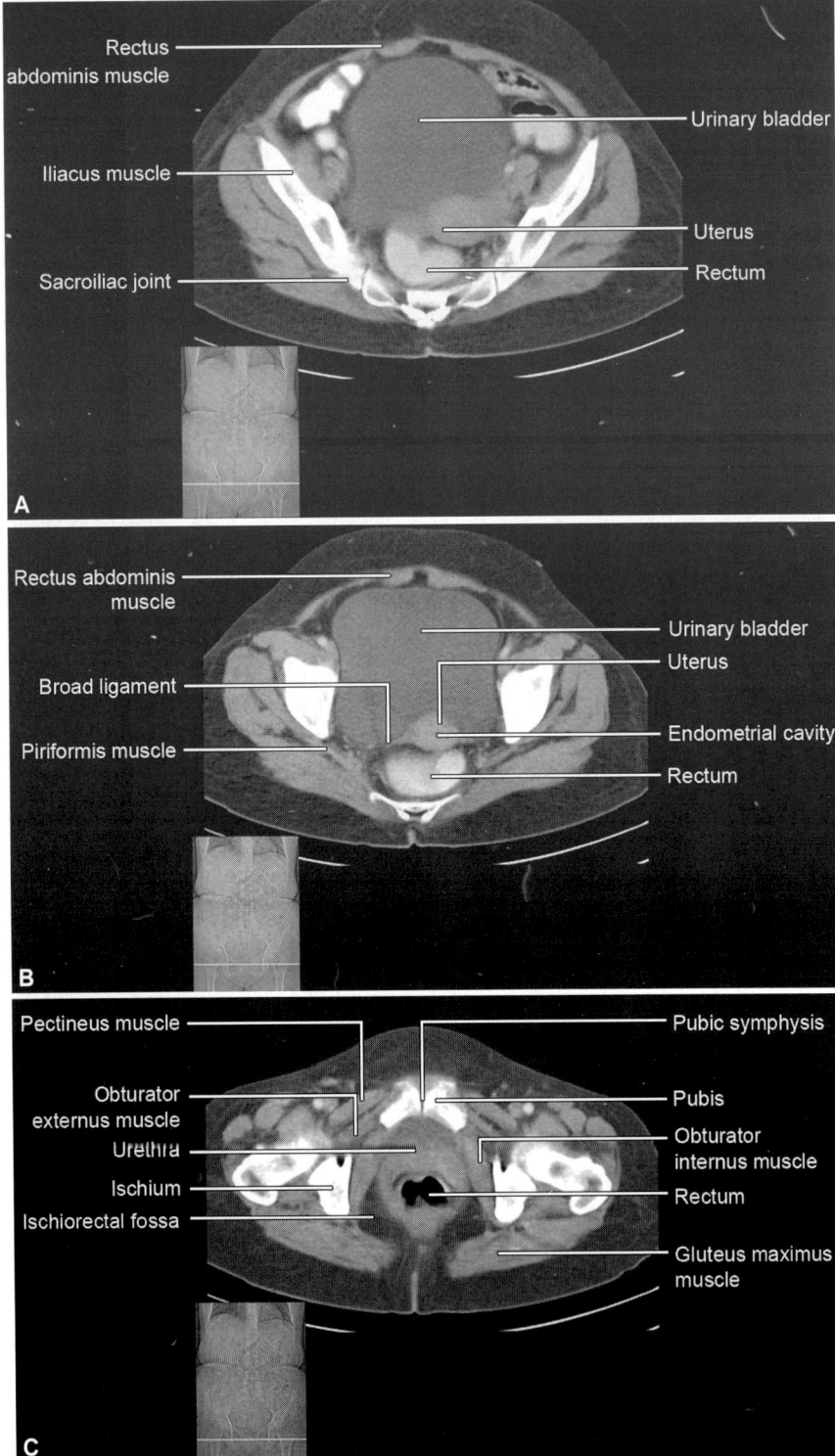

Figs 3A to C

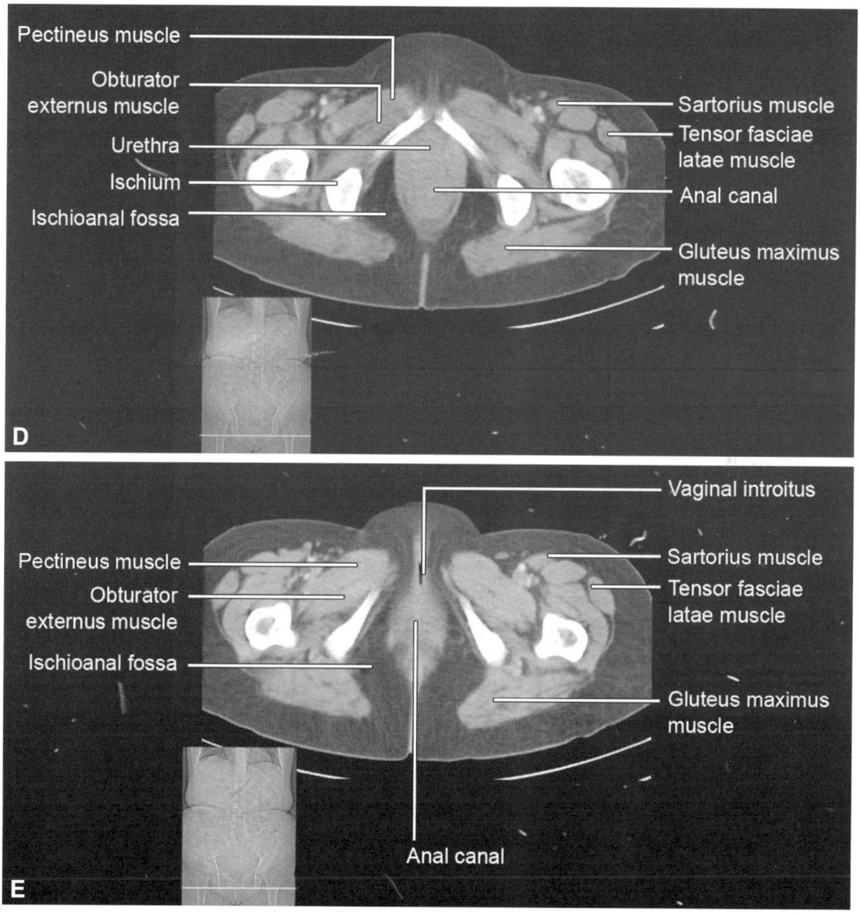

CT Anatomy: Abdomen and Pelvis

Figs 3D and E

Figs 3A to E Axial CT sections of female pelvis

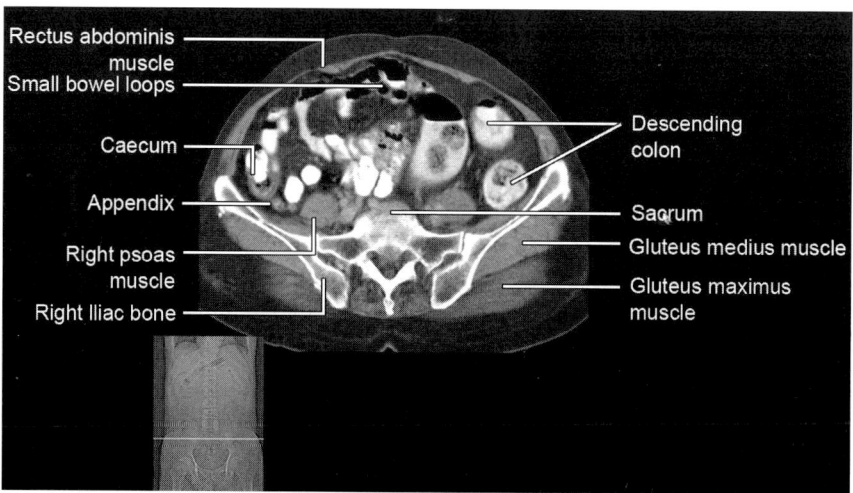

Fig. 4 Axial CT section showing appendix

When two folds of peritoneum connect a portion of bowel to the retroperitoneum it is known as mesentery. Ventral mesentery gives rise to falciform ligament, gastrohepatic ligament and hepatoduodenal ligament. Dorsal mesentery gives rise to gastrophrenic ligament, gastropancreatic ligament, phrenicocolic ligament, gastrosplenic ligament, splenorenal ligament and gastrocolic ligament. Dorsal mesentery also forms the small bowel mesentery and transverse as well as sigmoid mesocolons.

Omentum is a structure connecting stomach to an additional structure. Lesser omentum is formed by combination of hepatoduodenal and gastrohepatic ligament. Greater omentum is an inferior continuation of gastrocolic ligament and is composed of four layers of peritoneum resulting from double reflection of dorsal mesogastrium.

Anterior right subhepatic space located posterior to porta hepatis communicates with lesser sac through epiploic foramen also known as foramen of Winslow.

UROGENITAL SYSTEM

- Kidneys arise from metanephros (of mesodermal origin) at fourth week of intrauterine life. Bladder, urethra and prostate are formed from urogenital sinus.
- Adult kidneys have a span of 7–12 cm. Renal arteries arise from abdominal aorta at the level of L1-L2 vertebrae and then divide into following five segmental branches: apical, anterior superior, anterior inferior, posterior and basilar (Figs 2K to P).
- Renal arteries can be multiple, aberrant, accessory and even supplementary. Single or multiple renal veins can exist (Fig. 2N).
- Retroperitoneum is the space between parietal peritoneum extending from diaphragm to pelvic brim and fascia transversalis.
- Adrenal glands (suprarenal glands) are situated on the top of kidneys and are 3 cm long and 1 cm thick (Fig. 2L).
- Average size of testis is 2.5 × 3.0 × 3.5 cm. Epididymis has a head, body and a tail.
- Spermatic cord consists of testicular artery, cremasteric artery, pampiniform plexus of veins, vas deferens, nerves and lymphatics.
- Gonadal artery arises from ventral surface of aorta slightly below the origin of renal arteries. Occasionally it can arise from renal artery.
- Gonadal veins drain in the IVC or renal vein on right and in the renal vein on left.
- Prostate has a normal size of 2.5 × 2.8 × 3.0 cm (Fig. 5). It is composed of an outer part having a central and peripheral zone and an inner part made of periurethral and transitional zone.
- Male urethra is 15–20 cm long and has a posterior part composed of prostatic urethra and membranous urethra. The anterior part of urethra is composed of bulbar and penile urethra.

Female urethra is 2.5–5 cm long (Figs 3C and D).

Adult uterus is 6–9 cm long, 2.5–4 cm anteroposterior and 3–4.5 cm transverse in dimension. Endometrium is the innermost zone of uterus (Figs 3A and B). Serosa is the outermost zone. Myometrium is the middle layer. CT scan usually does not show them separately.

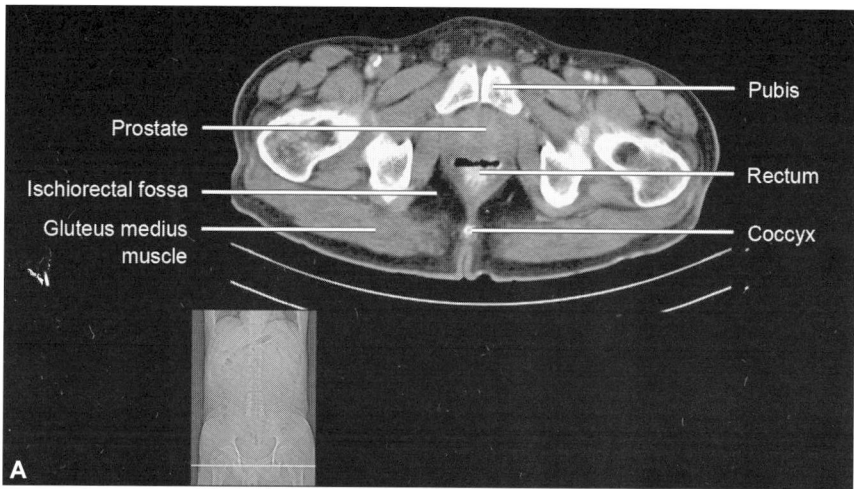
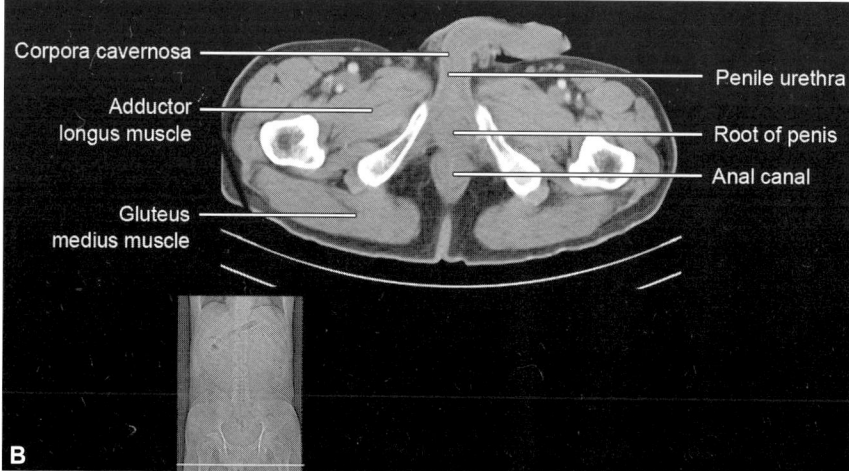

Figs 5A and B Axial CT sections of male pelvis

Fallopian tubes arise from upper and the outer aspect of uterus, and extend between the folds of broad ligament towards the pelvic side walls to open just above and anterior to ovaries located in ovarian fossa on each side.

Pelvic spaces formed due to relationship between urinary bladder, uterus and rectum are:
- Recto uterine pouch of Douglas
- Uterovesicle pouch
- Rectovesicle recess.

Important Pelvic ligaments in relation to uterus are:
- Broad ligament—between uterus and pelvic sidewalls
- Round ligament—between uterus and labia majora
- Cardinal ligament/Mackenrodt's ligament—between cervix and fascia of obturator internus
- Uterosacral ligament—between uterus and sacrum
  Adult ovaries measure 0.5–1.5 cm × 1.5–3.0 cm × 2–3 cm.

SECTION 1

Esophagus

1. Hiatus Hernia
2. Esophageal Carcinoma
3. Leiomyomatosis of Esophagus

CASE 1

Hiatus Hernia

CASE

A 43-year-old male with history of epigastric pain and burning sensation over a period of 2–3 months was referred to department of radiology for CT thorax.

Radiological Findings on CT Examination

Contrast enhanced axial CT image (Fig. 1) at the level of heart shows presence of portion of fundus of the stomach which is seen anterior and left lateral to the

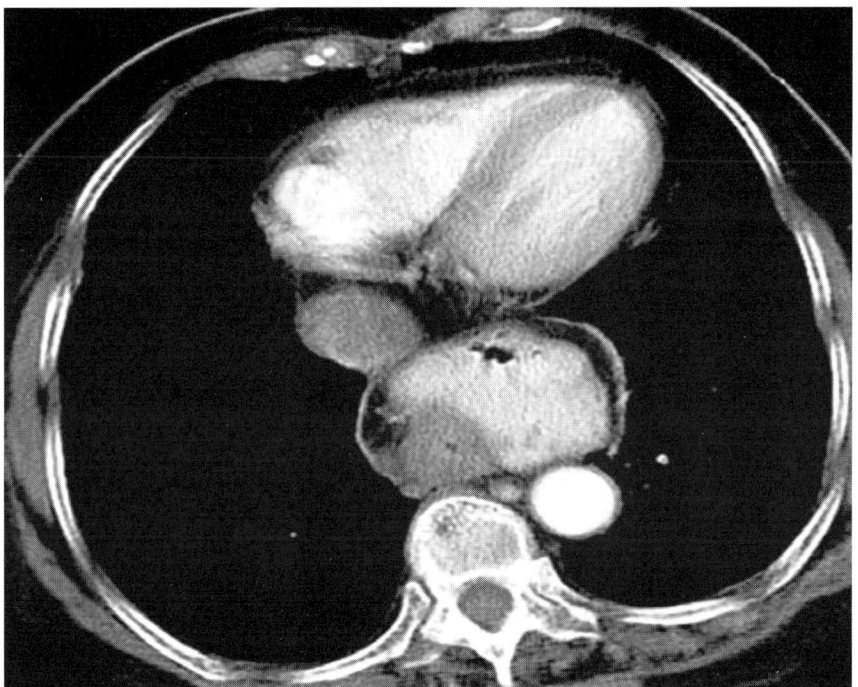

Fig. 1

esophagus. This is suggestive of upward displacement of the stomach through the esophageal hiatus suggestive of hiatus hernia.

Comments and Explanation

Hiatus hernia is a condition in which there is upward displacement of the gastroesophageal junction and/or the portion of the stomach through the esophageal hiatus. Embryologic development of the diaphragm is a complex process; a number of defects result in a variety of possible congenital hernias through the diaphragm. A hernia may occur through a congenitally large esophageal hiatus; however, acquired hernias through the esophageal hiatus are more common.

Opinion

Hiatus hernia.

Clinical Discussion

Hiatus hernias are classified either as sliding hernias, paraesophageal (rolling) hernias or mixed. Sliding hiatus hernias are the most common and account for 95% of the cases. In sliding hernia the gastroesophageal (GE) junction is >2 cm above the diaphragm. In rolling hernia the GE junction is below diaphragm but the gastric fundus protrudes through the hiatus. In mixed variety characters of both the types of hernia are seen. Most hiatus hernias are found incidentally, and they are usually discovered on routine chest radiographs or CT. Symptomatic, patients may experience heartburn, dyspepsia, or epigastric pain. Rarely, the patient may present with recurrent chest infections resulting from aspiration of gastric contents. A paraesophageal or, rarely, a sliding hiatal hernia may present with a volvulus or strangulation. Paraesophageal hernias are particularly likely to incarcerate and cause symptoms of intermittent epigastric pain. Barrett esophagus is commonly associated with hiatal hernia; patients with Barrett esophagus may present with reflux symptoms or dysphagia. Large incarcerated hiatal hernias may slowly bleed so that patients present with iron deficiency anemia, rather than reflux symptom. Other complications include peptic esophagitis from reflux, discrete marginal ulcer and strictures.

CASE 2

Esophageal Carcinoma

CASE

A 65-year-old male presented to the department of radiology with dysphagia.

Radiological Findings on CT Examination

CT scan abdomen shows circumferential wall thickening involving the gastroesophageal junction extending up to the fundus and lesser curvature of stomach (Figs 1A to C). Fat planes between this lesion and left lobe of liver is lost.

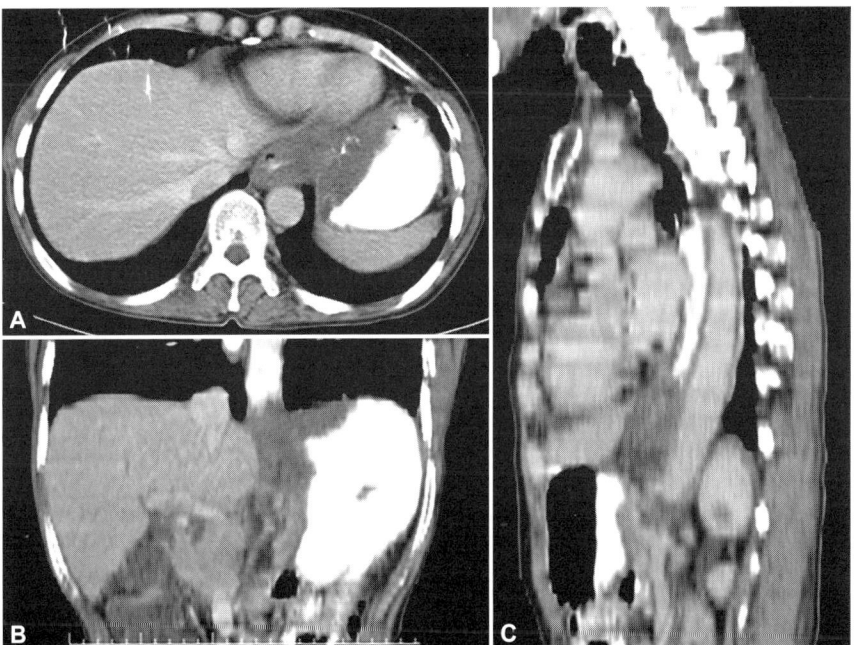

Figs 1A to C

Comments and Explanation

Carcinoma of the esophagus is relatively uncommon. Patients present with increasing dysphagia, initially to solids and progressing to liquids as the tumor increases in size. Barium is the initial study and shows irregular stricture, prestricture hold-up of contrast and ulceration. CT shows eccentric circumferential wall thickening >5 mm, dilated fluid filled esophageal lumen proximal to an obstructing lesion. Contrast-enhanced CT plays an important role in the staging of esophageal carcinoma. CT helps in determining the extent of the local tumor; invasion of mediastinal structures, involvement of supraclavicular, mediastinal, or upper abdominal lymph nodes; and distant metastases. The CT criteria for local invasion include loss of fat planes between the tumor and adjacent structures in the mediastinum, and displacement or indentation of other mediastinal structures. Aortic invasion is suggested if 90° or more of the aorta is in contact with the tumor or if there is obliteration of the triangular fat space between the esophagus, aorta, and spine adjacent to the primary tumor. A tracheobronchial fistula or tumor extension into the airway lumen is a definite sign of tracheobronchial invasion. Displacements of the trachea or bronchus, or indentation of the posterior wall of the trachea or bronchus by the tumor, have also proved accurate in predicting tracheobronchial invasion. Pericardial invasion is suspected if pericardial thickening, pericardial effusion, or indentation of the heart with loss of the pericardial fat plane is seen. Positron emission tomography (PET) has become a standard oncologic imaging modality. PET is useful not only for the primary detection of tumor and metastases but also for the further characterization of abnormalities discovered by using other imaging modalities.

Opinion

Esophageal carcinoma.

Clinical Discussion

Esophageal cancer is the third most common gastrointestinal malignancy. As with all other tumors, the outcome for patients with esophageal cancer is strongly associated with the stage at initial diagnosis. More than 90% of esophageal cancers are either squamous cell carcinomas (SCCs) or adenocarcinomas. SCCs are evenly distributed between the middle and lower esophagus, whereas approximately three-fourths of all adenocarcinomas are found in the distal esophagus. Esophageal cancer is notorious for its aggressive behavior; it may invade local, regional, or distant structures by various pathways, including direct extension, lymphatic spread, and hematogenous metastasis. CT, endoscopic US, and PET all play important roles in the staging of patients with esophageal cancer. CT is a good initial screening modality for determining whether the patient may undergo resection or has distant metastases. The most common sites of metastases include liver, lungs, bones, adrenal glands, kidneys, and brain. PET is useful for assessing distant metastases as well as restaging after neoadjuvant therapy.

CASE 3
Leiomyomatosis of Esophagus

CASE

A 25-year-old female patient with history of dysphagia was referred to radiology department for CT scan thorax and abdomen.

Radiological Findings on CT Scan Examination

CT scan thorax and abdomen (Figs 1A to C) show diffuse circumferential thickening of mid and lower esophageal wall extending up to the gastro-esophageal junction and fundus of stomach. The entire eosophageal lumen is dilated. Fat planes with the adjacent structures are preserved.

Gross specimen of the esophagus reveals circumferential thickening of esophagus (Fig. 1D). Cut surface of the esophageal specimen shows abnormal muscular thickening with intact mucosa (Fig. 1E). This turned out to be esophageal leiomyomatosis on histopathologic examination.

Comments and Explanation

Esophageal leiomyomatosis is a rare clinical entity characterized by proliferation of smooth muscle cells in the esophageal wall, causing circumferential thickening. Although it can occur at any age, it is more common in children and young adults, and is more common in women. In pediatric patients, the usual age at presentation is between 10 and 14 years. Chest X-ray, barium swallow, endoscopy, CT scan, magnetic resonance imaging and EUS are commonly used diagnostic modalities. A chest X-ray shows a mediastinal mass or widening of the mediastinum. Barium swallow study reveals dilatation of the upper esophagus and smooth tapering of the distal esophagus with decreased or absent esophageal peristalsis, mimicking the appearance of achalasia. It is not easy to differentiate these two entities, though the narrowed segment in achalasia is usually shorter than in leiomyomatosis. The CT scan usually shows circumferential thickening of the esophageal wall that extends to the cardia. This feature differentiates esophageal leiomyomatosis from achalasia. It should also be differentiated from diffuse circumferential thickening of the esophageal musculature that may occur

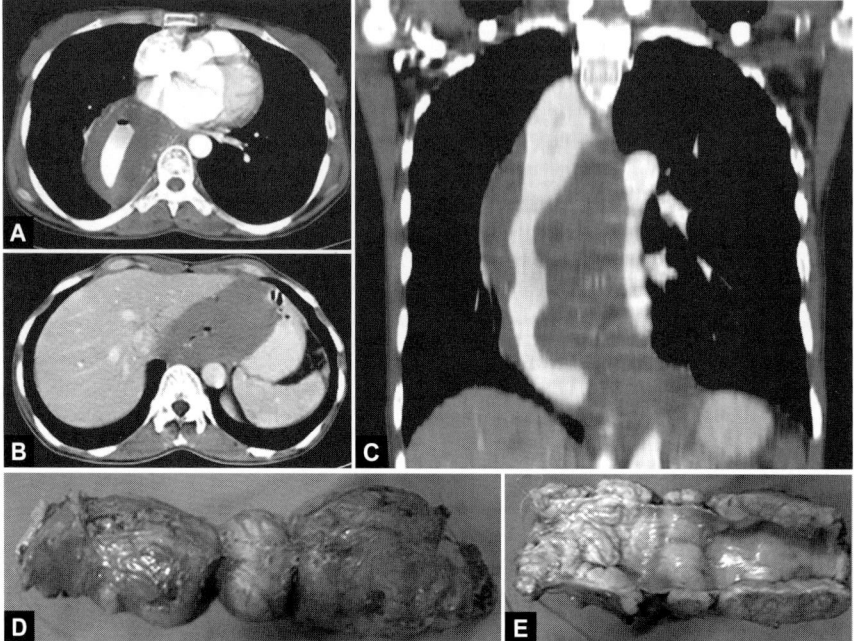

Figs 1A to E *(For color version D and E, see plate 2)*

in neuromotor functional disorders. In addition it must be distinguished from leiomyoma, which is a focal, encapsulated lesion and a true neoplasm. Another differential diagnosis of circumferential wall thickening of esophagus is malignant tumor. Upper endoscopy also is helpful because it may show irregularity of the wall due to submucosal lesions that are mostly covered by normal mucosa.

Opinion

Esophageal leiomyomatosis.

Clinical Discussion

Esophageal leiomyomatosis is a rare, benign condition in which neoplastic proliferation of smooth muscle causes marked circumferential thickening of the esophageal wall, most commonly in the distal esophagus. Patients develop symptoms because of encroachment of the lumen of the esophagus by thickened and hypertrophied musculature. The most common presentation is dysphagia for a long duration, regurgitation, dyspepsia, cough, dyspnea and weight loss. Because of its rarity, the preoperative diagnosis is usually difficult. Early evaluation with CT may be valuable in demonstrating the intramural location and nature of the disease and differentiating this entity from achalasia and other causes of dysphagia. The narrowed segment in patients with achalasia tends to be shorter. No sarcomatous change in leiomyomatosis of the esophagus has been reported. However, surgical removal of the lesion is nearly always indicated in symptomatic patients. Surgical methods depend on the extent of the lesion. An esophagectomy or esophagogastrectomy is usually curative and prognosis is good.

SECTION 2

Diaphragm

4. Eventration
5. Eventration of Diaphragm with Duplication of Inferior Vena Cava

CASE 4

Eventration

CASE

A 15-year-old male with acute pain in abdomen was referred to the department of radiology for CT scan chest and abdomen.

Radiological Findings on CT Examination

Axial contrast-enhanced computed tomography (CECT) at chest level and sagittal reconstruction of chest and abdomen shows eventration of right hemidiaphragm with right kidney migrating into chest at D8 vertebral level under the diaphragm (Figs 1A and B). Barium enema examination shows redundancy of the colon with ascending colon and cecum extending into the right hemithorax underlying the right hemidiaphragm (Fig. 1C). Upper GIT study (not in the figure) demonstrated the stomach in normal position with duodenojejunal flexure on the right side as a part of malrotation of right gut.

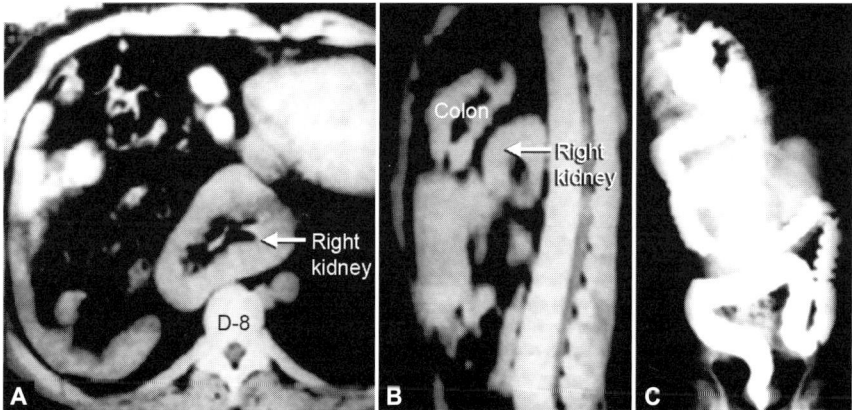

Figs 1A to C

Comments and Explanation

Elevation of a single hemidiaphragm is usually secondary to adjacent pleural, pulmonary, subphrenic disease or due to phrenic nerve palsy. Rarely it is related to an intrinsic weakness of the diaphragm. In eventration weakened diaphragmatic muscles results in the upward displacement of abdominal contents but its incidence with malrotation of midgut is generally not seen. Occasionally it is associated with superior renal ectopia as the kidney continues to migrate beyond the normal renal fossa during development and ends up in the thorax as seen in this case.

Opinion

Eventration of diaphragm.

Clinical Discussion

Diaphragmatic eventration refers to an abnormal contour of the diaphragmatic dome and is typically due to incomplete muscularization of the diaphragm with a thin membranous sheet replacing normal diaphragmatic muscle. Over a period this region stretches and on inspiration does not contract normally. Usually it is thought to be congenital. Commonly seen on right side. Elevation of the affected portion of the diaphragm is usually seen as a smooth hump on the normal contour of the hemidiaphragm.

CASE 5

Eventration of Diaphragm with Duplication of Inferior Vena Cava

CASE

A 20-year-old female with history of vomiting and acute pain in abdomen was referred to the department of radiology for CT scan abdomen and pelvis.

Radiological Findings on CT Examination

CT abdomen shows elevated right dome of diaphragm which lies at the level of D6, large and small bowel loops are seen closely abutting it (Figs 1A to E).

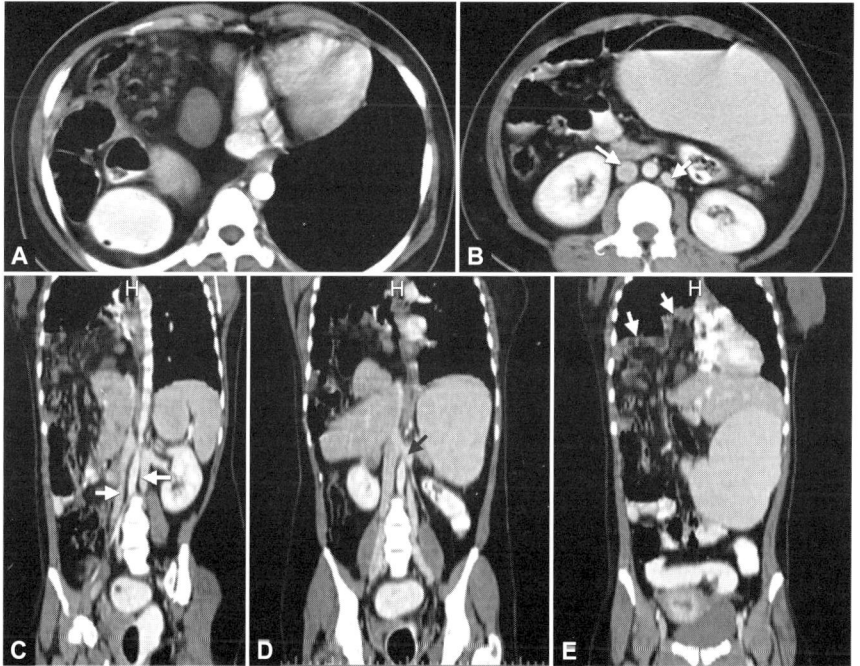

Figs 1A to E

Duplication of IVC (white arrows) is seen as an incidental finding. In this the left common iliac vein ascends as left IVC and the left renal vein (black arrow) drains into it which crosses anterior to the aorta and joins the right IVC (Figs 1C and D). The right IVC is larger in diameter than the left IVC (Fig. 1B).

Comments and Explanation

Diaphragmatic eventration refers to an abnormal contour of the diaphragmatic dome and is due to incomplete muscularization of the diaphragm with a thin membranous sheet replacing normal diaphragmatic muscle. This has been discussed in Case 04.

In double IVC, both left and right supracardinal veins persist. Duplication of inferior vena cava is a rare vascular anomaly, but this abnormality needs to be recognized, especially in association with renal anomalies like crossed fused ectopia. The left common iliac vein ascends as duplicated left IVC and usually drains into the left renal vein, which then crosses anterior to the aorta and joins the right IVC in a normal fashion, i.e. incomplete double IVC. It is possible that the left IVC does not drain into the left renal vein, but after receiving the left renal vein it continues with a major preaortic trunk that travels obliquely and empties into the right IVC, i.e. complete double IVC. The complete duplication of IVC could be subclassified into three types: Type I or major duplication: comprises two bilaterally symmetrical trunks and a preaortic trunk of the same caliber. Type II or minor duplication: comprises two bilaterally symmetrical trunks, but smaller than the preaortic trunk. Type III or asymmetric duplication: comprises small left IVC, larger right IVC and even larger preaortic trunk.

Opinion

Eventration of diaphragm with duplication of IVC.

Clinical Discussion

An important differential for IVC duplication is transposition of IVC, in which IVC continues on left side of aorta, where as in duplication, IVC is seen on both sides of aorta.

SECTION 3

Stomach

6. Gastrointestinal Stromal Tumor
7. Gastric Malignanacy

CASE 6

Gastrointestinal Stromal Tumor

CASE

A 45-year-old female patient with history of lump in right hypochondrium was referred to radiology department for CT scan.

Radiological Findings on CT Scan

CT scan abdomen (Figs 1A and B) show a well defined soft tissue density mildly enhancing lesion in lesser sac between the posterior margin of left lobe of liver and lesser curvature of stomach. The lesion is infiltrating the lesser curvature of stomach. In lower CT sections (Figs 1C and D) show a large exophytic lobulated heterogeneously enhancing soft tissue density lesion involving the duodenum and adjacent small bowel loops. It shows central cystic/necrotic component with air fluid level. Both these lesions represent stromal tumors.

Figure 1B shows an ill defined heterogeneously enhancing lesion in segment VII of right lobe of liver representing metastases.

Comments and Explanation

The term stromal tumor was coined in 1983 by Clark and Mazur for smooth muscle neoplasm of the gastrointestinal tract (GIT). Gastrointestinal stromal tumors (GIST) are nonepithelial tumors arising from the interstitial cells of Cajal. The clinical manifestations of GISTs depend on the location and size of the tumors and are often nonspecific. Common symptoms include early satiety, indigestion, bloating, vague abdominal pain, and a palpable mass. Occasionally, gastrointestinal bleeding occurs with tumors involving the mucosa. Because of these nonspecific clinical symptoms and the exophytic growth of the tumors, GISTs are often not detected until late in their progression

Opinion

Gastrointestinal stromal tumor (GIST).

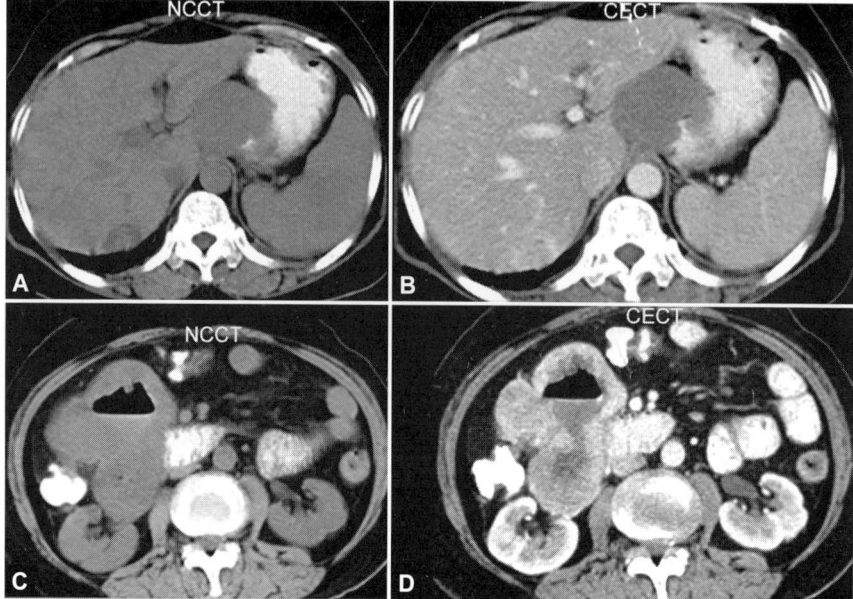

Figs 1A to D

Clinical Discussion

Gastrointestinal stromal tumors (GIST) can arise anywhere in the GI tract, including the mesentery, omentum, and rarely retroperitoneum. Since most of these tumors are submucosal in location, they usually attain a large size without causing bowel obstruction. Many of these tumors have an exophytic component as they arise from the muscularis propria. CT is the imaging modality of choice for diagnosis and staging of GISTs at initial presentation and for monitoring the disease during and after treatment. GISTs are typically large, hypervascular, enhancing masses on contrast-enhanced CT scans and often appear heterogeneous due to necrosis, hemorrhage, or cystic degeneration. Fistulization to the gastrointestinal lumen are also common features of GISTs. The masses usually displace adjacent organs and vessels. Direct invasion of the adjacent structures is seen with advanced disease. Sometimes it can be difficult to identify the origin of the mass because of its large size and prominent extraluminal location. Calcification is uncommon. Differential includes esophageal leiomyoma which is most commonly in the esophagus but is rare in the remainder of the gastrointestinal tract. Most metastases of GISTs involve the liver and peritoneum by hematogenous spread and peritoneal seeding, respectively and less commonly metastases are found in the soft tissue, lungs, and pleura. GISTs metastasizing to the lymph nodes are extremely rare.

CASE 7

Gastric Malignanacy

CASE

A 50-year-old male with complaints of hematemesis and weight loss was referred to radiology department for CT scan abdomen.

Radiological Findings on CT Scan

Computed tomography (CT) scan abdomen (Fig. 1A) shows marked thickening of the entire gastric wall with narrowing of gastric lumen in a case of gastric lymphoma.

Other Cases of Carcinoma Stomach

Figure 1B CT scan abdomen in right lateral recumbent position of the patient carcinoma of the pylorus shows circumferential thickening of pylorus with the growth extending into antrum and duodenum. Prepyloric lymph node is seen (arrow).

Figure 1C shows homogeneously enhancing circumferential thickening of almost the entire stomach wall in a case of carcinoma of stomach. Few enlarged lymph nodes are also present.

Figure 1D shows ascites and bilateral ovarian deposits (Krukenberg tumor) in a previously operated case of carcinoma stomach.

Comments and Explanation

Gastric malignancy continues to be one of the leading causes of cancer related death. An important development in the epidemiology of gastric carcinoma has been the recognition of the association with *Helicobacter pylori* infection. Adenocarcinoma is by far the most common gastric malignancy, representing over 95% of malignant tumors of the stomach. The remaining malignant tumors include lymphoma, sarcoma, metastasis, and so on. CT is currently the staging modality of choice because it can help identify the primary tumor, assess for local spread, and detect nodal involvement and distant metastases. Detection

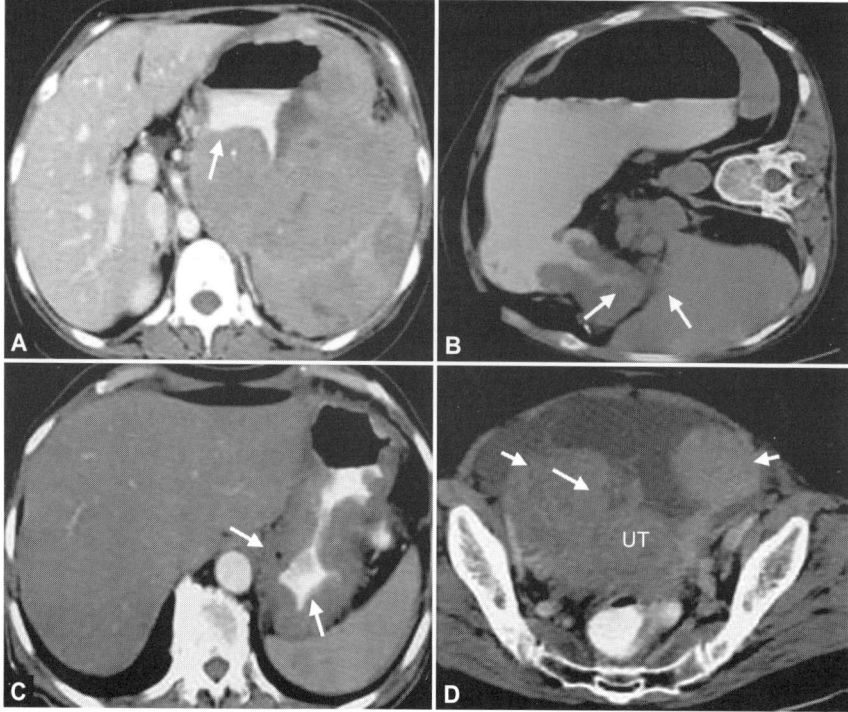

Figs 1A to D

of gastric carcinoma is improved by using thin-section sequences and helical or multidetector-row CT. CT can show polypoid mass with or without ulceration or focal wall thickening with mucosal irregularity. In linitus plastica the stomach wall is diffusely thickened. The underlying cause is usually scirrhous adenocarcinoma with diffuse submucosal infiltration, leading to thickening and rigidity to the stomach wall. Metastases in cases of gastric carcinoma occur along peritoneal ligaments and also to local lymph nodes. Lymphangitic spread may occur to lungs. Hematogenous spread occurs in liver, adrenals, ovaries and bones.

Opinion

Gastric Carcinoma.

Clinical Discussion

Gastric cancer is rare before 40 years of age, and its incidence peaks in the seventh decade of life. Carcinoma stomach often produces no specific symptoms when it is superficial although up to 50% of patients may have nonspecific gastrointestinal complaints such as dyspepsia. Some patients may present with anorexia and weight loss as well as abdominal pain that is vague and insidious in nature. Nausea, vomiting, and early satiety may occur with bulky tumors that obstruct the gastrointestinal lumen or infiltrative lesions that impair stomach distension. Endoscopy is regarded as the most sensitive and specific diagnostic method in patients suspected of harboring gastric cancer. Endoscopy allows direct visualization of tumor location, the extent of mucosal involvement, and biopsy for tissue diagnosis. But radiological methods are often the initial examination that raises suspicion for gastric carcinoma, besides being used in the staging of the disease. Double-contrast barium examinations have a sensitivity of 90–95% in gastric cancer detection. Computed tomography (CT) scanning, magnetic resonance imaging (MRI), and endoscopic ultrasonography (EUS) are used in the staging, but not usually in the primary detection of gastric cancer.

SECTION 4

Duodenum

8. Carcinoma Duodenum

CASE

8   Carcinoma Duodenum

CASE

A 60-year-old male presented to the department of radiology with abdominal pain and distension.

Radiological Findings on CT Examination

Axial post contrast CT images of abdomen (Fig. 1A) shows heterogeneously enhancing mass lesion in second part of the duodenum with surrounding fat stranding and loss of fat planes between the lesion and adjacent structures. Two small hypodense lesions are seen in right lobe of liver (Fig. 1B). These findings suggest duodenal carcinoma with hepatic metastases.

Comments and Explanation

Adenocarcinoma is the most common primary malignant neoplasm of the duodenum. It represents 0.3% of all gastrointestinal malignancies. It accounts for 50–70% of small bowel adenocarcinomas occurring either in the duodenum or proximal jejunum. There is an increased risk of carcinoma in patients with familial adenomatous polyposis and adenomas in the duodenum. Small bowel carcinomas may be associated with increased incidence of primary malignancies at other locations. Disease progression may be assessed by lymph node involvement and spread to the liver, spleen, lungs.

Opinion

Carcinoma duodenum with hepatic metastases.

Clinical Discussion

In general upper abdominal pain and weight loss are the symptoms, and usually they are not suggestive of ulcer. In the late phases of the disease a variety of symptoms and signs have been reported, commonly those of developing high

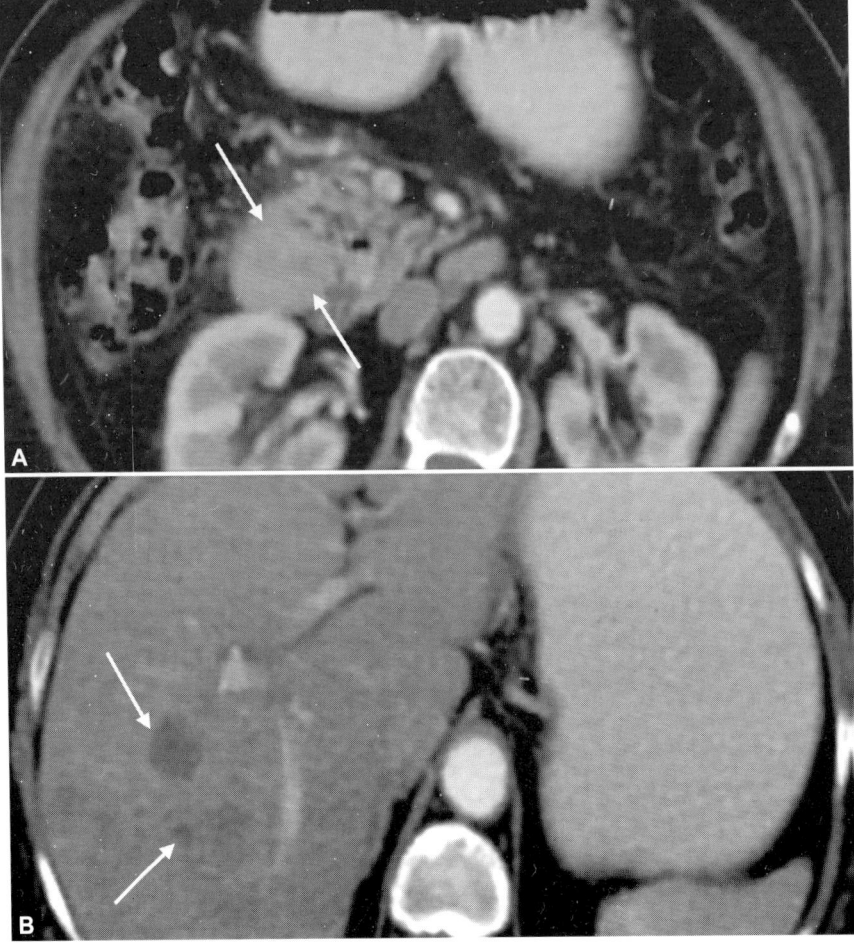

Figs 1A and B

intestinal obstruction and jaundice, hematemesis, melaena, and occult blood in the stool. A variety of other findings, such as low back pain and alteration in bowel habit, have also been described. Grossly duodenal carcinomas have napkin ring appearance or polypoidal fungating mass. Patients with familial adenomatous polyposis and Gardeners syndrome are considered to have a higher likelihood of developing duodenal cancer. Patients who have duodenal polyps without a predisposing family history are also at an increased risk. Ultrasonography can diagnose and assess vascularity of larger lesions but the smaller tumors (<2 cm) may not be detected. CT is the modality of choice for staging of the disease by identifying primary tumor, assessing local, nodal and distant spread. Duodenal adenocarcinoma is associated with a delayed diagnosis and poor prognostic and survival outcomes due to nonspecific clinical presentation. Metastasis, poor tumor differentiation, increased depth of spread and pre-existing Crohn's disease are associated with poor prognosis.

SECTION 5

Small Bowel

9. Small Bowel Obstruction
10. Ileocecal Lymphoma
11. Small Bowel Gastrointestinal Stromal Tumor
12. Angiodysplasia of Jejunum
13. Ileal Carcinoma
14. Pneumatosis Intestinalis
15. Midgut Volvulus

CASE 9
Small Bowel Obstruction

CASE

A 40-year-old male presented to the department of radiology with severe pain in abdomen since two days.

Radiological Findings on CT Examination

Abdominal radiograph (Fig. 1A) shows radially arranged dilated small bowel loops which is confirmed on the coronal reconstructed CT image of abdomen. Dilatation and abrupt cut off of bowel loops is well seen on the reconstructed CT image (Fig. 1B). These findings are suggestive of small bowel obstruction.

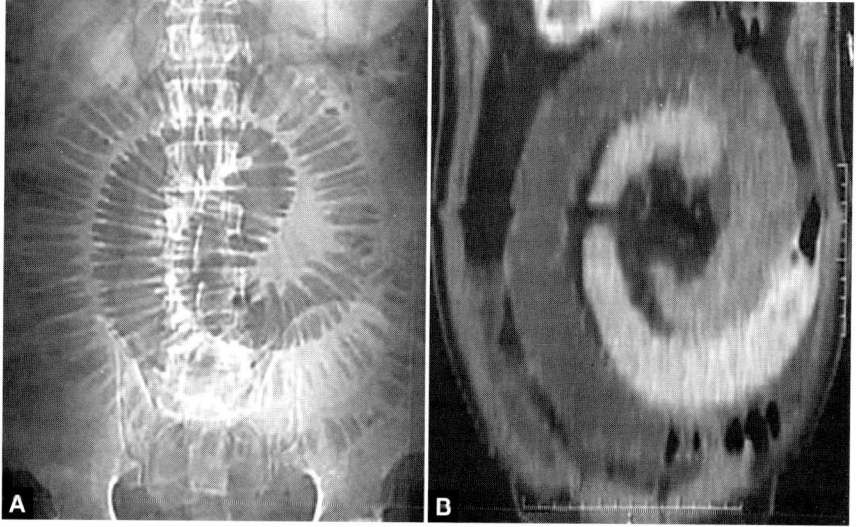

Figs 1A and B

Comments and Explanation

Small bowel obstruction is most commonly due to mechanical obstruction, leading to dilated bowel loops and multiple air fluid levels. If an obstruction cuts off the blood supply to the intestine, the condition is called strangulation. Strangulation occurs in nearly 10 to 20% of cases with small-intestinal obstruction. Usually, strangulation results when part of the intestine becomes trapped in an abnormal opening (strangulated hernia), volvulus, or intussusception. Gangrene can develop in as few as 6 hours. With gangrene, the intestinal wall is necrosed, usually causing rupture, which leads to peritonitis, shock, and, if untreated, death.

Opinion

Small Bowel obstruction.

Clinical Discussion

A small-bowel obstruction is caused by a variety of pathologic processes. The leading cause of small bowel obstruction in industrialized countries is postoperative adhesions (60%), followed by malignancy, Crohn disease, and hernias. Intestinal obstruction usually causes cramping pain in the abdomen, accompanied by bloating and anorexia. Vomiting is common with small-intestinal obstruction but is less common and begins later with large-intestinal obstruction. Complete obstruction causes severe constipation, whereas partial obstruction may cause diarrhea. With strangulation, pain may become severe and steady. Fever is common and is particularly likely if the intestinal wall ruptures. In most of the cases abdominal radiograph will be helpful since it will show dilated bowel loops and multiple air fluid levels. In complicated cases CT abdomen will give the correct diagnosis. CT will help to determine cause and complications due to obstruction.

CASE 10

Ileocecal Lymphoma

CASE

A 60-year-old male with history of abdominal distension and weight loss was referred to the Department of Radiology for CT scan abdomen.

Radiological Findings on CT Examination

Figures 1A and B show a heterogeneously enhancing soft tissue density lesion involving the cecum, ileocecal (I-C) junction and terminal ileum. Anteriorly fat planes between this lesion and anterior abdominal wall are lost.

Gross specimen (Fig. 1C) shows a solid mass lesion involving the cecum, I-C junction and terminal ileal loop. This turned out to be Non-Hodgkin's lymphoma on histopathologic examination.

Comments and Explanation

The small bowel is the second most frequent site of gastrointestinal tract involvement by lymphoma. Most cases of small bowel lymphoma are due to Non-Hodgkin's lymphoma. Lymphomas constitute approximately one-half of all primary malignant small bowel tumors. The ileum is the most common site of occurrence, the duodenum the least frequent. CT appearance of lymphoma is variable. The typical appearance can be classified as aneurysmal, constrictive, nodular and ulcerative infiltration. Definitive diagnosis is based on histopathological examination from biopsy of the lesion.

Opinion

Ileocecal Non-Hodgkin's Lymphoma.

Clinical Discussion

Non-Hodgkin lymphomas (NHLs) are tumors originating from lymphoid tissues, mainly of lymph nodes. These tumors may result from chromosomal

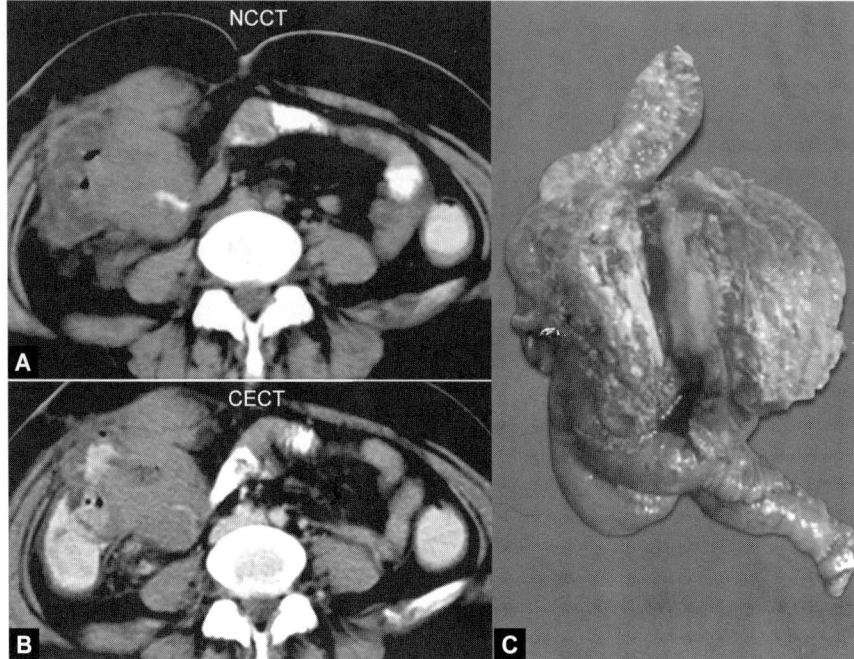

Figs 1A to C *(For color version C, see plate 2)*

translocations, infections, environmental factors, immunodeficiency states, and chronic inflammation. The clinical manifestations of NHL vary with such factors as the location of the lymphomatous process, the rate of tumor growth, and the function of the organ being compromised or displaced by the malignant process. Signs and symptoms of low-grade lymphomas include the following. Peripheral adenopathy which is painless and can spontaneously regress. Primary extranodal involvement. Bone marrow involvement is frequent may be associated with cytopenias. Fatigue and weakness more common in advanced-stage disease.

Primary lymphoma criteria include:
- Confinement of disease to a small bowel segment
- Only regional lymphadenopathy
- No hepatic or splenic involvement except by direct tumor extension
- No palpable or mediastinal lymphadenopathy
- Normal peripheral blood smear and bone marrow biopsy.

CASE 11

Small Bowel Gastrointestinal Stromal Tumor

CASE

A 45-year-old male presented to the department of radiology with lump in left hypochondriac region.

Radiological Findings on CT Examination

Axial and coronal reconstructed CT images of abdomen (Figs 1A and B) show a well defined lobular heterogenously enhancing mass lesion arising from the small intestine. The lesion is exophytic and no evidence of obvious obstruction noted. Findings are suggestive of gastrointestinal stromal tumor (GIST).

Comments and Explanation

Gastrointestinal stromal tumors are believed to arise from the interstitial cells of Cajal with 95% staining positive for CD117 (c-KIT) and 70% for CD34.

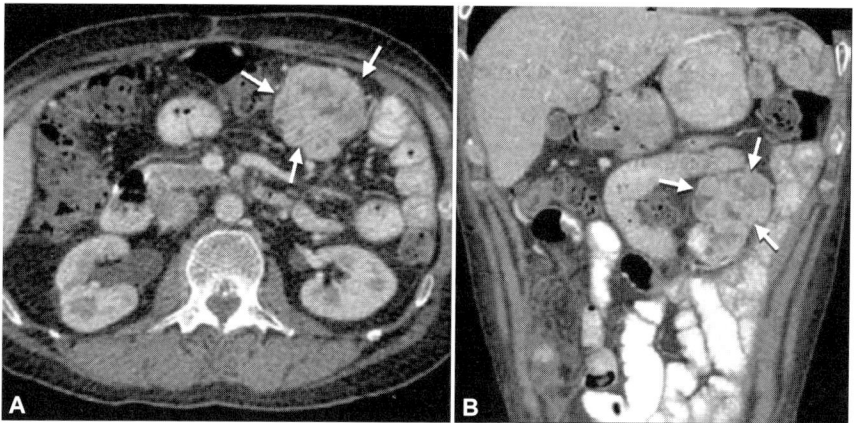

Figs 1A and B

The majority of GIST have a uniform appearance, falling into one of three categories: spindle cell, epithelioid cell, and mixed cell. Because most of these tumors are submucosal in location, they usually attain a large size without causing bowel obstruction by the time of diagnosis. Many of these tumors have an exophytic component as they arise from the muscularis propria. The enhancement pattern can vary from homogenously enhancing to heterogenously enhancing, with or without ulceration.

Opinion

Gastrointestinal stromal tumor (GIST).

Clinical Discussion

The clinical findings vary depending on the location and size of the tumor at presentation. If the tumor is small, it may be only an incidental finding during radiological imaging or surgery for some other cause, whereas a large exophytic lesion may present as an abdominal mass due to its large size. Lesions in the stomach, small bowel, or colon may present with gastrointestinal bleed in the form of hematemesis, malena, or occult blood in stools; alternatively, there may be abdominal pain, nausea, and vomiting. An esophageal GIST most commonly presents with dysphagia. GISTs generally occur with equal frequency in both the sexes. They are common in the fourth and fifth decades of life. GISTs can arise anywhere along the GIT. In the esophagus, leiomyomas are more common than GIST; however, in the stomach, small intestine, and colon, GISTs are the most common mesenchymal tumors. For localizing the organ of origin and defining the extent of the mass, 64-row multidetector computed tomography (MDCT) with multiplanar reformations may be helpful. Metastases from GIST commonly occur to the liver and peritoneal cavity via hematogenous spread and peritoneal seeding and occasionally occur to soft tissues, lungs, and pleura. Tumors to be considered in the differential diagnosis of GIST include adenocarcinoma, lymphoma, peritoneal carcinomatosis, carcinoid and metastases. Imatinib is a new chemotherapeutic agent used in the treatment of GIST. It is a molecularly targeted tyrosine kinase receptor blocker. Response to imatinib is usually good, with improved long-term survival. The imaging features in patients showing response to imatinib include decrease in the density of the lesion, reduction in enhancement, and reduction in the number of nodules and number of vessels.

CASE 12

Angiodysplasia of Jejunum

CASE

A 70-year-old male with history of chronic per rectal bleeding and anemia was referred to the department of radiology for CT scan abdomen.

Radiological Findings on CT Examination

Contrast enhanced CT abdomen coronal and sagittal reconstructions (Figs 1A and B) show evidence of an intensely enhancing lesion involving the wall of jejunum. Rest of the bowel loops and mesentery appear normal.

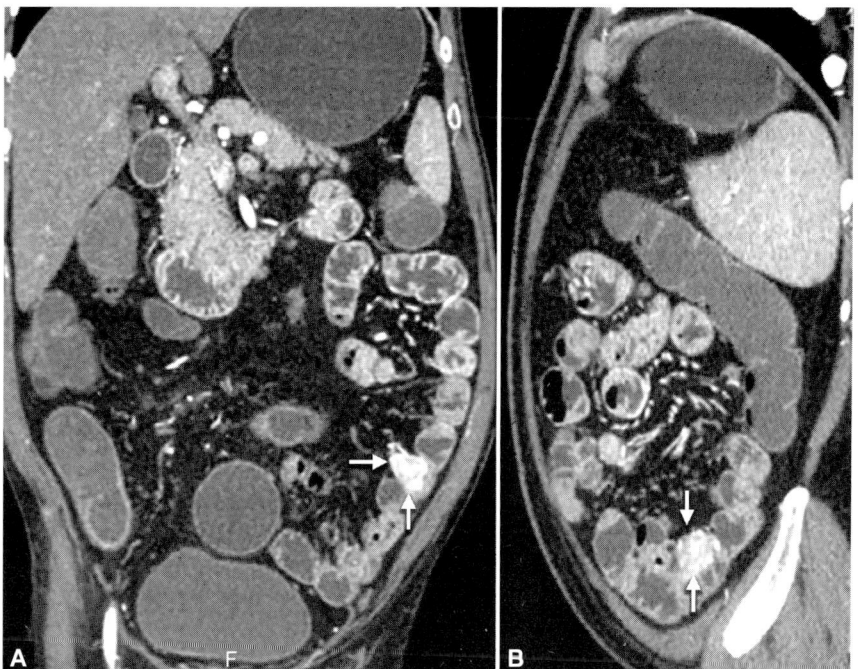

Figs 1A and B

Comments and Explanation

Angiodysplasia is a condition of unknown etiology in which microvascular abnormalities are found in mucosa and submucosa of the bowel wall. The lesion is predominantly found in caecum and right side of the colon. It is frequently associated with acute or chronic intermittent blood loss. It is not associated with family history or any other vascular abnormality. Endoscopy and angiography are the most common methods of diagnosing angiodysplasia. Other diagnostic tools include double-contrast barium enema, CT angiography, and radionuclide scanning.

Opinion

Angiodysplasia of jejunum.

Clinical Discussion

Most patients found to have angiodysplasia are older than 60 years. No racial predilection is there and it is seen in equal frequency in males and females. Many patients with angiodysplasia are asymptomatic, and the lesions are incidentally found during screening with colonoscopy. Hemorrhage from angiodysplasia is episodic. Angiography will show a cluster of small arteries during the arterial phase along the antimesenteric border of the colon. There will be accumulation of contrast material in vascular spaces and intense opacification of the bowel wall during the capillary phase followed by early opacification of dilated draining veins that persists late into the venous phase. Clinical presentation and physical examination are related to GI bleeding or its consequences. Angiodysplasia can be seen in more than one location in GI tract. Depending upon the site of the lesion the presentation varies. Patients having lesion in upper GI tract may present with hemetemesis and if lesion is in lower GI tract then malena is commoner presentation. Malena occurs in at least one fourth of patients with colonic bleeding. Spontaneous cessation of bleeding (occurring in 90% of patients) is the rule for angiodysplastic lesions located in any part of the GI tract.

CASE 13

Ileal Carcinoma

CASE

A 70-year-old male presented to the department of radiology with chronic constipation and weight loss.

Radiological Findings on CT Examination

Axial and coronal reconstruction contrast enhanced CT images of abdomen (Figs 1A and B) show an enhancing mass in terminal ileum. The mass is seen to narrow

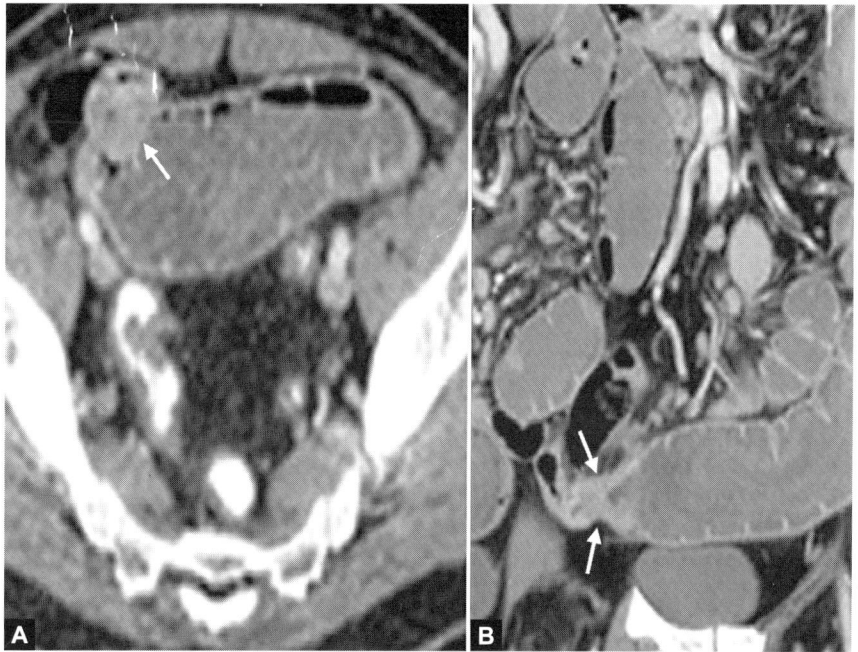

Figs 1A and B

the lumen and there is evidence of dilatation of bowel proximal to the narrowing. There is evidence of adjacent fat stranding and lymphadenopathy. Findings are suggestive of ileal carcinoma.

Comments and Explanation

Primary neoplasms of the small intestine are very rare, comprising approximately 1.6–6% of all tumors of the gastrointestinal tract, 60% of these tumors are malignant and are most commonly seen in the 5th and 6th decades of life. Adenocarcinoma is the most common malignant tumor of the small intestine. It presents as enhancing mass lesion which can be either polypoidal or napkin ring. Also it can present with obstruction and prestenotic dilatation of the bowel loops.

Opinion

Ileal adenocarcinoma.

Clinical Discussion

In general, small-bowel cancer prevalence is lower in Asia and in less industrialized countries than in western countries. Men have higher rates of all types of small bowel cancer than women. Most small bowel tumors are asymptomatic until the late stages of disease. Symptoms when they occur include nonspecific abdominal pain, weight loss, diarrhea, and constipation. Signs related to a complication like bleeding, obstruction, or perforation may also be observed. Various genetic disorders are also associated with an increased incidence of small bowel tumors like Peutz Jhegers syndrome—hamartomatous polyps, Gardner's syndrome—adenoma, adenocarcinoma. Plain-film radiography can show a dilated proximal jejunum and air-fluid levels if obstruction is present. A barium examination will reveal annular narrowing or stricture formation, filling defects or polypoid masses. The most typical radiological manifestation is a narrowed segment with features of mucosal destruction, also known as the "apple core" sign. CT may show an eccentric focal mass or a circumferential irregular thickening of the small bowel wall. CT is the most effective technique for studying retroperitoneal tumor extent and liver metastases. MRI may also help to demonstrate tumor extension and metastatic disease.

CASE 14

Pneumatosis Intestinalis

CASE

A 40-year-old male patient with history of pain in abdomen since 7 days was referred to radiology department for CT scan abdomen.

Radiological Findings on CT Scan

CT scan abdomen (Fig. 1) shows multiple air pockets in multiple segments of small bowel wall.

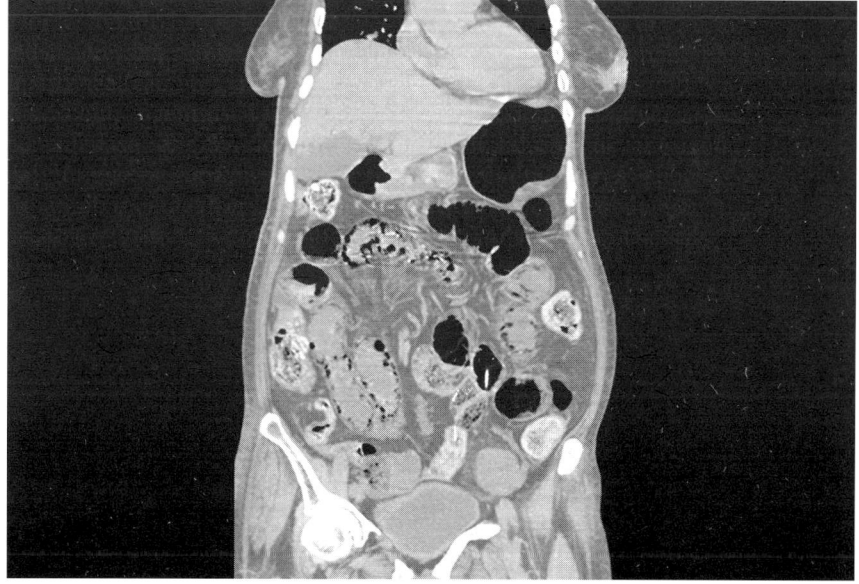

Fig. 1

Comments and Explanation

Gas in the bowel wall, or pneumatosis intestinalis, can occur as a primary isolated entity or in conjunction with diseases of the gastrointestinal or respiratory systems. In primary pneumatosis no disease process is present and it occurs mainly in adults and involves the colon. It requires no treatment and resolves spontaneously except in rare cases of hemorrhage, obstruction, or perforation. Secondary pneumatosis intestinalis more commonly involves the small bowel and is associated with a wide variety of conditions that affect the gastrointestinal systems such as ischemia, obstruction, infection (particularly necrotizing enterocolitis in infants), peptic ulcer disease, inflammatory bowel diseases, endoscopy, colonoscopy, or surgery. Imaging modality of choice is CT, which will show intramural gas, portal venous gas and pneumoperitoneum. Depending on etiology bowel wall/mesenteric edema may be seen. Lung windows are used to look for gas collections. CT with IV contrast is used to assess mesenteric vascular patency.

Opinion

Pneumatosis intestinalis.

Clinical Discussion

Pneumatosis intestinalis is seen in the setting of intestinal ischemia and infarction. Other etiologies like medications (steroids, chemotherapy, immunosuppressants) and autoimmune disorders (SLE, scleroderma) cause increased mucosal permeability which can lead to pneumatosis. Any form of mucosal disruption like trauma, ulcers, irritable bowel disease, endoscopy and surgical anastomoses can cause pneumatosis intestinalis. Clinical presentation varies from abdominal pain/distention, fever, gastrointestinal bleed to sepsis. Gas in the bowel wall in the neonatal period is diagnostic of necrotising enterocolitis.

CASE 15

Midgut Volvulus

CASE

A 25-year-old male patient with complaints of intermittent pain in abdomen since one month was subjected to CT scan abdomen.

Radiological Findings on CT Examination

There is twisting of mesentery and few small bowel loops around the superior mesenteric artery (Figs 1A and B). Jejunal loops appear edematous and most of them are seen occupying the right side of abdomen (Fig. 1C). There is reversal of superior mesenteric artery (SMA) and superior mesenteric vein (SMV) relationship, i.e. SMV is to the left of SMA (arrows Fig. 1C). Cecum and ileocecal junction is seen in midline in lower abdomen (arrow Fig. 1D).

Comments and Explanation

The twisting of small bowel is normally prevented because of the normal broad fixation of the mesentery. Narrow base of the mesentery allows the small bowel and mesentery to twist and wrap around itself to create a distinctive 'whirlpool' appearance on CT scan. This pattern was first described by Fisher. Abnormal orientation of the superior mesenteric artery and superior mesenteric vein relationship is not entirely diagnostic of malrotation, it can be seen as a normal variant in some patients and a proportion of patients with malrotation may have a normal SMA-SMV relationship.

Opinion

Midgut volvulus.

Clinical Discussion

Derivatives of the midgut include the distal half of 2nd, 3rd and 4th part of duodenum, jejunum, ileum, cecum, appendix, ascending colon and proximal

Figs 1A to D

two-thirds of the transverse colon. These structures are supplied by the superior mesenteric artery, which also serves as the axis of midgut rotation. Midgut volvulus is a complication of malrotation in which clockwise twisting of the bowel around the superior mesenteric artery (SMA) axis occurs because of the narrowed mesenteric attachment. In 20% it is associated with duodenal atresia and annular pancreas. Congenital malrotation of the midgut often presents within the first month of life. In adults recurrent episodes of colicky abdominal pain, with vomiting over a period of months or years are typical. Ultrasound can show distended proximal duodenum. Superior mesenteric vein to the left of SMA. Thick-walled bowel loops inferior to duodenum and to the right of spine associated with free peritoneal fluid. The degree of twisting can change due to natural movement of bowel. Severe volvulus causes obstruction of SMV and SMA which leads to bowel necrosis. Color Doppler shows mesenteric vessels moving clockwise with caudal movement of transducer, this is called as clockwise whirlpool sign. The CT whirlpool sign describes the swirling appearance of bowel and mesentery twisted around the SMA axis.

SECTION 6

Appendix

16. Acute Appendicitis
17. Appendicular Abscess

CASE 16

Acute Appendicitis

CASE

A 40-year-old female with history of pain in right iliac fossa, fever, vomiting since 3 days was referred to the department of radiology for CT abdomen and pelvis.

Radiological Findings on CT Examination

Axial post contrast CT images show an enlarged long appendix with its tip in midline in infraumbilical region. Its wall shows enhancement (Fig. 1A). There is periappendiceal fat stranding and a small loculated collection adjacent to the tip of appendix (arrow) (Fig. 1B).

Comments and Explanation

Appendicitis essentially means inflammation of the appendix. It is a very common condition in general radiology practice and is a major cause of abdominal surgery in young patients. Appendicitis is typically caused by obstruction of the appendiceal lumen, with resultant build up of fluid, secondary infection, venous congestion, ischemia and necrosis. Ultrasound should be the investigation of choice in young patients since it lacks ionizing radiation. The technique used is

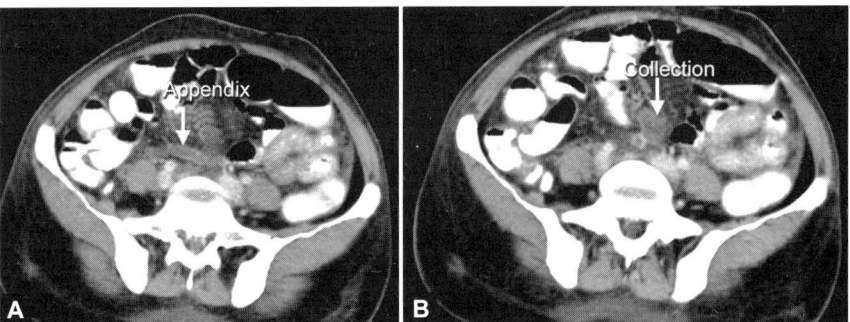

Figs 1A and B

known as graded compression and uses the linear probe, with gradual increasing pressure exerted to displace the normal overlying bowel gas. Appendix is seen as a blind ending noncompressible, tubular aperistaltic structure with diameter > 6 mm. It shows a target appearance on transverse section. On Doppler there is increased circumferential flow. Appendicolith is seen as an echogenic focus with distal shadowing within the lumen of appendix. Thickening of adjacent bowel wall, fluid collections, hypoechoic mass indicate perforation of appendix. Due to its high sensitivity and specificity, CT is becoming the preferred imaging modality for suspected acute appendicitis since it is less operator dependent than USG. Concerns have grown over the possible adverse effects on patients from exposure to radiation from CT scanning. Low-dose abdominal CT is preferred as it allows for a 78% reduction in radiation exposure compared to traditional abdominopelvic CT. It shows features like, dilated appendix with distended lumen (>6 mm diameter), thickened and enhancing wall, thickening of the caecal apex (caecal bar sign), periappendiceal inflammation, including stranding of the adjacent fat and thickening of the lateroconal fascia or mesoappendix and extraluminal fluid. Progression of the inflammatory process may lead to formation of sealed abscess. An abscess with a well-defined border usually indicates chronicity and the presence of air bubbles or air fluid levels inside indicates the presence of gas-forming organisms or communication of the abscess with the bowel.

Opinion

Appendicitis.

Clinical Discussion

Acute appendicitis is the most common surgical abdominal emergency. It is commonly seen in children and young adults with peak incidence in the 2nd to 3rd decades of life. Classically presentation consists of periumbilical pain (referred) which within a day or later localizes to Mc Burney's point and is associated with fever, nausea and vomiting. Patient may have leukocytosis. In most of the cases obstruction is important causative factor. Inflammation of the appendix results from obstruction of its lumen from fecaliths, foreign bodies, lymphoid hyperplasia, parasites, or tumors. The lumen of the appendix becomes obstructed, leading to increased intraluminal pressure resulting in inflammation, ischemia, and infection. The differential diagnosis of appendicitis is often a clinical challenge because appendicitis can mimic several abdominal conditions. Patients with many other disorders present with symptoms similar to those of appendicitis, such as the following pelvic inflammatory disease, ovarian cyst or torsion, mesenteric adenitis, diverticulitis, omental torsion, renal colic and ectopic pregnancy. Recognized complications of acute appendicitis include perforation, abscess formation and generalized peritonitis.

CASE 17

Appendicular Abscess

CASE

A 53-year-old male patient with history of fever and abdominal lump was subjected to CT abdomen and pelvis.

Radiological Findings on CT Examination

Figure 1B CT abdomen and pelvis coronal reconstruction image shows enlarged appendix with periappendiceal fat stranding. A loculated fluid collection with a peripherally enhancing wall is seen in right iliac fossa adjacent to the appendix. Air pocket is seen within it (Fig. 1A).

Comments and Explanation

Abscess formation is the most common complication of appendicitis. Plain radiograph may show free air, appendicolith in right iliac fossa and displacement

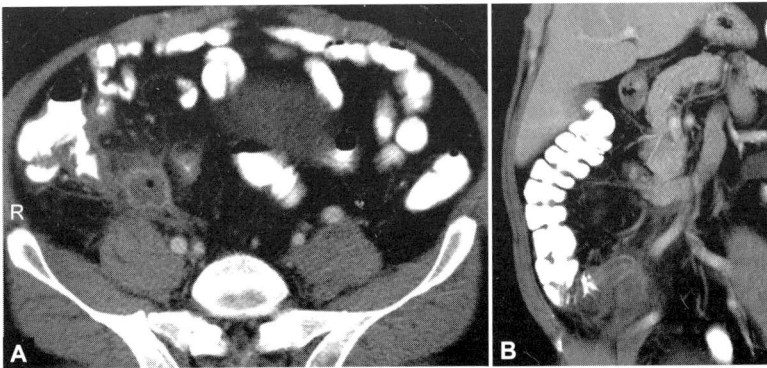

Figs 1A and B

of cecal gas. Small bowel obstruction pattern may be seen. Ultrasound is primary screening modality and may show hypoechoic fluid collection in the appendicular region which may be well circumscribed and rounded or ill-defined and irregular in appearance. Appendix may be visualized within the mass. CT is the examination of choice and may show fluid collection with peripherally enhancing wall with or without air within. Sometimes appendicolith may be seen.

Opinion

Appendicular abscess.

Clinical Discussion

An appendicular abscess is a complication of acute appendicitis. Patients with appendicular abscess usually have a history of severe colicky pain in the right lower abdomen (right iliac fossa) with a tender boggy swelling in this region. Other symptoms may include vomiting, constipation or less frequently, diarrhea. On examination the abdomen may be rigid and the swelling can be felt. When the appendix becomes inflamed (appendicitis), complications arise if the infection is not treated promptly. In some patients, appendicitis can lead to gangrene of appendix. In most of these patients the intestinal coils and omentum in the abdominal cavity tend to cover the inflamed gangrenous appendix. This forms an appendicular mass. The continuing suppurative process inside the appendicular mass can lead to the formation of an abscess. An abscess with a well-defined border usually indicates chronicity and the presence of air bubbles or air fluid levels inside indicates the presence of gas-forming organisms or communication of the abscess with the bowel. Patients with abscess larger than 4 cm size and high fever are usually managed with drainage of abscess.

SECTION 7

Colon

18. Intussusception
19. Nontoxic Megacolon
20. Sigmoid Diverticulitis
21. Abdominal Koch's
22. Carcinoma Sigmoid

CASE 18

Intussusception

CASE

A 30-year-old male patient came with history of pain in abdomen and vomiting and was referred to radiology department for CT scan abdomen.

Radiological Findings on CT Scan Examination

Contrast enhanced CT scan abdomen (Figs 1A and B) show intussusception involving the transverse colon. No evidence of proximal bowel dilatation. (Fig. 1A) shows classic bowel within bowel appearance of intussusception involving the transverse colon.

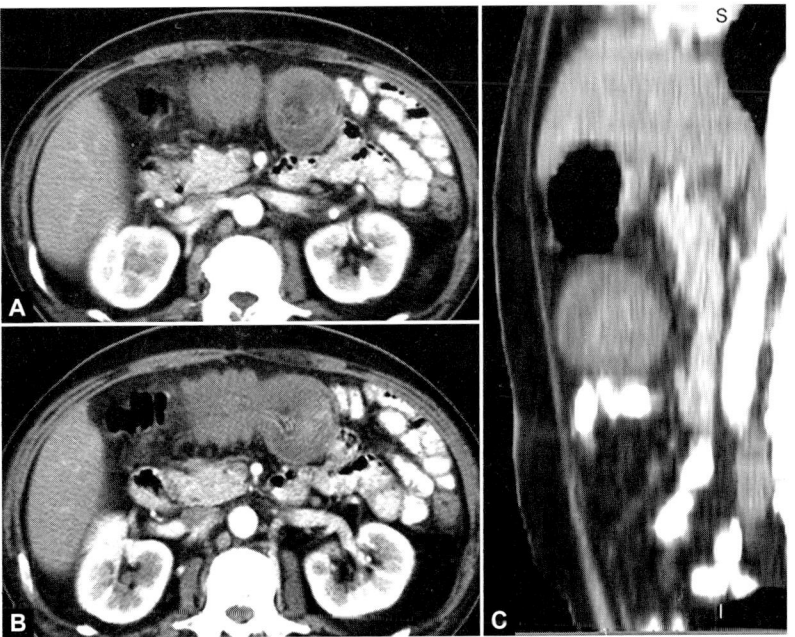

Figs 1A to C

Comments and Explanation

Intussusception involves the telescoping of a loop of bowel and its mesentery (intussusceptum) into the lumen of contiguous bowel (intussuscipiens) because of abnormal peristalsis related to a lead point mass. Intussusceptions are more common in children. Intussusception is more common in children and is the leading cause of bowel obstruction in this population. Intussusceptions in adults are uncommon. Majority of adult intussusceptions involve a lead point mass, two-thirds of which are neoplastic. Intussusceptions can be classified according to their location—enteroenteric (small bowel only), ileocolic (prolapse of terminal ileum into ascending colon), ileocecal (ileocecal valve or colon serves as the lead point) and colocolic (large bowel only).

Opinion

Colocolic intussusception.

Clinical Discussion

In children cyclical colicky abdominal pain, vomiting, currant jelly stools (diarrhea with mucus and blood) are the presenting features. Adults usually present with intermittent crampy abdominal pain over days to months or there can be acute obstruction with hours to days of abdominal distention, pain, and constipation. Rarely patient can present with a palpable abdominal mass. Plain radiographs are not sensitive or specific but can show soft tissue mass surrounded by a crescent of gas and evidence of distal small bowel obstruction. Barium enema is diagnostic and therapeutic. Barium is seen in the lumen of the intussusceptum and in the intraluminal space giving a coiled spring appearance. Ultrasound findings are (1) On transverse scan—"Doughnut sign" = concentric rings of alternating hypoechoic and hyperechoic layers (intussuscepiens) with central hyperechoic portion (mesentery of intussusceptum). (2) On longitudinal scan—"Sandwich, pseudo-kidney or hayfork sign" = layering of hypoechoic bowel wall and hyperechoic mesentery. Color Doppler demonstrates mesenteric vessels dragged between entering and returning wall of intussusceptum. Absence of blood flow within the intussusceptum suggests bowel necrosis. Presence of blood flow within the intussusceptum is a good predictor of reducibility. Abdominal CT is the most sensitive imaging modality for diagnosing intussusception. Three CT patterns of intussusception have been described and are thought to correspond to different stages of the process. They were initially described by Merine in 1987. The target appearance occurs when an intraluminal soft-tissue mass and eccentric fat density are seen as a result of the intussusceptum and the intussuscepting mesentery. This pattern usually corresponds to an early intussusception with only minimal obstruction, if any. These patients typically do not have signs of ischemia at pathology. The reniform pattern is described as peripheral high attenuation and lower attenuation centrally. This appearance is thought to result from a thickened bowel wall surrounding the intussusceptum, probably resulting from underlying ischemia. The sausage-shaped pattern results from alternating areas of low and high attenuation related to the bowel wall, mesenteric fat and fluid, intraluminal fluid, contrast material, or air. In adults with intussusception involving the colon, primary resection without reduction is recommended. Reduction increases the risk of intraluminal seeding or venous embolization of a possible tumor and can cause perforation and peritoneal soiling in cases of bowel ischemia. However, for transient, otherwise asymptomatic enteroenteric intussusceptions without a lead point, intervention is usually not necessary, as these frequently resolve spontaneously.

CASE 19

Nontoxic Megacolon

CASE

A 50-year-old male presented to the department of radiology with distension of abdomen.

Radiological Findings on CT Examination

Contrast enhanced CT images (coronal reconstruction and axial images at the level of pelvis) (Figs 1A and B) shows dilatation of left half of the transverse colon, descending colon and sigmoid colon. There is no evidence of pericolonic fat stranding or wall thickening which suggests that there are no inflammatory changes. The rectum is showing normal luminal diameter (Fig. 1C). Findings are suggestive of nontoxic megacolon.

Comments and Explanation

Megacolon is dilatation of colon > 6 cm. There is additional loss of haustral markings. If it is associated with inflammation of colon or signs of peritonitis, it is called as toxic megacolon. If there are no signs of inflammation and patient is only having distension of abdomen then it is non toxic megacolon. The etiology of this is not well understood. No large-scale studies have been conducted to determine incidence of acquired megacolon. However, once present, the approximate risk of a spontaneous perforation from nontoxic megacolon is 3%.

Opinion

Non toxic megacolon.

Clinical Discussion

Nontoxic megacolon is defined as severe dilatation of a segment or the entire colon unaccompanied by signs or symptoms of colon toxicity. Mechanical factors (volvulus, anastomosis, diverticulosis, carcinoma) are responsible for the

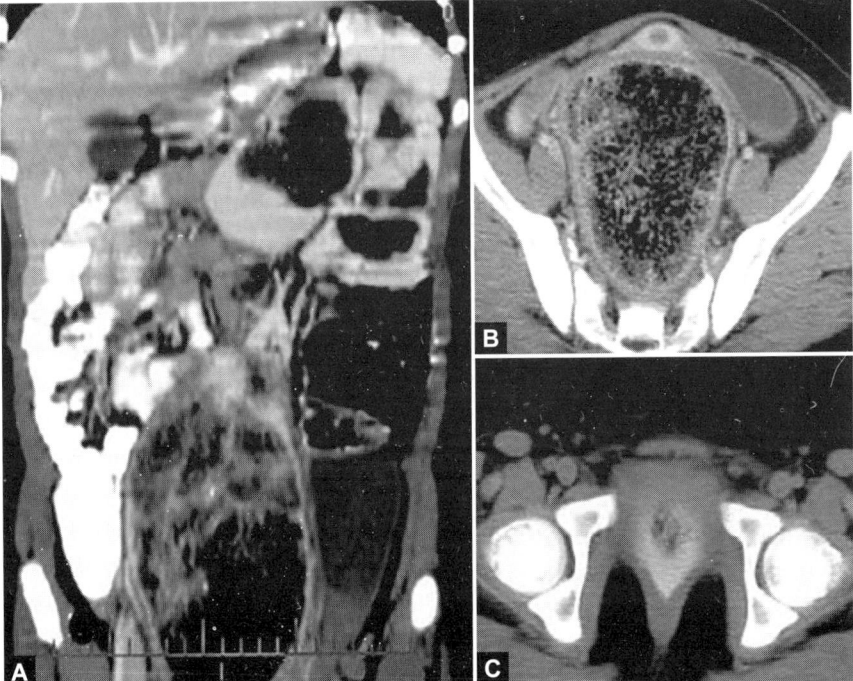

Figs 1A to C

nontoxic megacolon. It is seen sometimes secondary to acute pseudo-obstruction (Ogilive's syndrome, pancolonic megacolon, acute myxedemic ileus). The approximate risk of a spontaneous perforation from nontoxic megacolon is low. Colonoscopy should be considered as the initial treatment for nontoxic megacolon prior to surgical intervention. Colonoscopic decompression can successfully treat most of the pseudo-obstruction cases. However, in the cases of obstruction due to volvulus, surgical intervention is necessary. Barium studies should be avoided, due to the risk of perforation in these cases.

CASE 20

Sigmoid Diverticulitis

CASE

A 50-year-old male with complaints of pain in left iliac fossa since 4–5 days was referred to the department of radiology.

Radiological Findings on CT Examination

Post contrast axial CT image (Fig. 1) shows evidence of multiple air filled outpouchings involving the sigmoid colon suggesting multiple diverticuli.

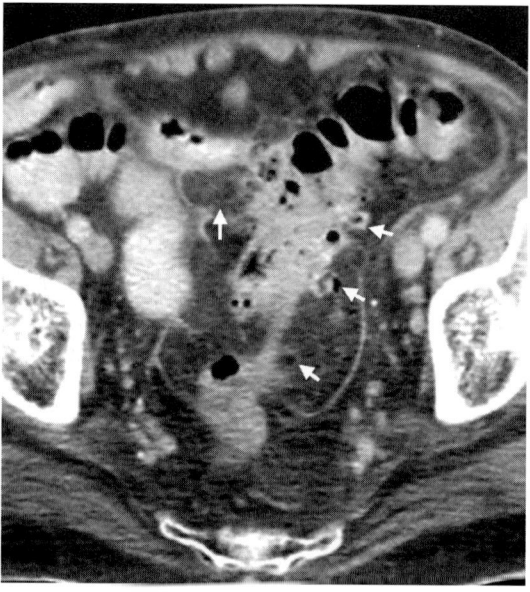

Fig. 1

There is thickening of the walls of these outpouchings and it shows contrast enhancement. Also there is surrounding fat stranding. All these findings suggest inflammation of these mentioned diverticuli suggestive of sigmoid diverticulitis.

Comments and Explanation

Mucosal and submucosal herniation through the muscular layer of colon gives rise to the diverticulum. It is commonly seen in the region of sigmoid colon. Inflammatory changes of these diverticuli give rise to diverticulitis. Estimated to occur in 10–15% of people with diverticulosis.

Opinion

Sigmoid diverticulitis.

Clinical Discussion

Diverticulitis is the most common complication of colonic diverticulosis. Most commonly appear in the sigmoid colon. Obstruction at neck of colonic diverticula by stool, inflammation, or food particles leads to bacterial overgrowth, vascular compromise and microperforation which in turn lead to pericolic inflammation. Symptoms of diverticulitis usually begin in the left iliac fossa with unremitting pain and accompanying tenderness. An ill defined mass may also be palpable representing the inflammatory phlegmon. On CT there is pericolic stranding, often disproportionately prominent compared to the amount of bowel wall thickening and segmental thickening of the bowel wall. Also there is enhancement of the colonic wall. Complications include fistula formation, abscess formation, adhesions, and pneumoperitoneum. Surgery is the treatment option for severe cases of sigmoid diverticulitis.

CASE 21

Abdominal Koch's

CASE

A 30-year-old male presented with fever, pain in abdomen and weight loss. Patient was referred to radiology department for CT scan abdomen and pelvis.

Radiological Findings on CT Examination

Figures 1A to C are axial post contrast images of abdomen. Figure 1A shows mesenteric fat stranding and lymphadenopathy. Colonic wall thickening is seen

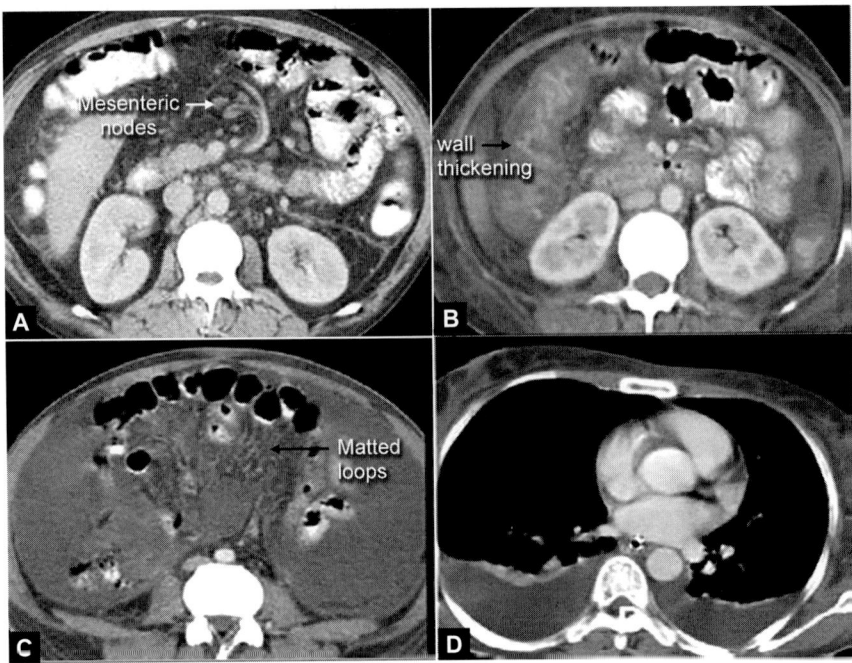

Figs 1A to D

in Fig. 1B. Figure 1C shows matted bowel loops. Figure 1D is axial post contrast image of thorax showing bilateral pleural effusions. All these findings indicate abdominal tuberculosis.

Comments and Explanation

Gastro-intestinal tuberculosis (GI TB) is a major health problem in many underdeveloped countries. A recent significant increase has occurred in developed countries, especially in association with HIV infection. It is a form of chronic infection. It may affect peritoneum, mesentery, bowel, liver, spleen, pancreas. The imaging findings depend upon the organ involvement and virulence of the organism. On ultrasound (USG) pathologic lymph nodes may appear as discrete nodular structures or appear as conglomerated masses. At CT affected nodes may have low attenuation values or soft tissue density. On contrast enhanced CT, they have typical peripheral enhancement with central nonenhancing areas. This pattern reflects significant central liquefactive or caseous necrosis and perinodal highly vascular inflammatory reaction. Homogeneous nodal enhancement or calcifications may also be seen. Peritoneal involvement is most commonly caused by rupture of an infected lymph node into the peritoneal cavity. Hematogenous or lymphatic seeding may also occur. USG shows the presence of free or loculated fluid, often with multiple mobile strands of fibrin and echogenic debris. On CT, ascites has high attenuation values due to the high protein content of the fluid. CT may also show regular or nodular peritoneal and mesenteric thickening with increased mesenteric vascularity. Thickened peritoneum usually shows contrast enhancement. Omental involvement may appear as omental nodules, diffuse infiltration and thickening. Omental cake may be seen. Bowel shows wall thickening. On CT, the most common findings of intestinal involvement are circumferential wall thickening of the cecum and terminal ileum and asymmetric thinking of the ileocecal junction. Associated pulmonary infection can be depicted by pleural effusion, pulmonary cavitary lesions and nodular opacities on CT Chest.

Opinion

Abdominal tuberculosis.

Clinical Discussion

Clinical features of intestinal TB include abdominal pain, weight loss, anemia, and fever with night sweats. Patients may present with symptoms of obstruction, right iliac fossa pain, or a palpable mass in the right iliac fossa. Hemorrhage and perforation are recognized complications of intestinal TB, although free perforation is less frequent than in Crohn's disease. The peritoneum and ileocecal region are commonly involved in majority of the cases by hematogenous spread or through swallowing of infected sputum from primary tubercular infection. The pulmonary tuberculosis may be apparent in about half of these cases. The ileum is more commonly involved than the jejunum. Ileocecal involvement is seen in 80–90% of patients with GI TB. This feature is attributed to the abundance of lymphoid tissue (Peyer's patches) in the distal and terminal ileum. Barium studies, CT scan, invasive procedures and serological tests now can help in timely diagnosis and early institution of treatment of such cases so as to reduce morbidity and mortality from this curable but potentially lethal disease. The treatment of abdominal tuberculosis is on the same lines as for pulmonary tuberculosis.

CASE 22

Carcinoma Sigmoid

CASE

A 70-year-old male presented with painless bleeding per rectum and was referred to Department of Radiology for CT scan abdomen.

Radiological Findings on CT Examination

Axial post contrast CT image at the level of pelvis shows circumferential irregular intraluminal growth in the distal sigmoid colon that turned out to be carcinoma (Fig. 1).

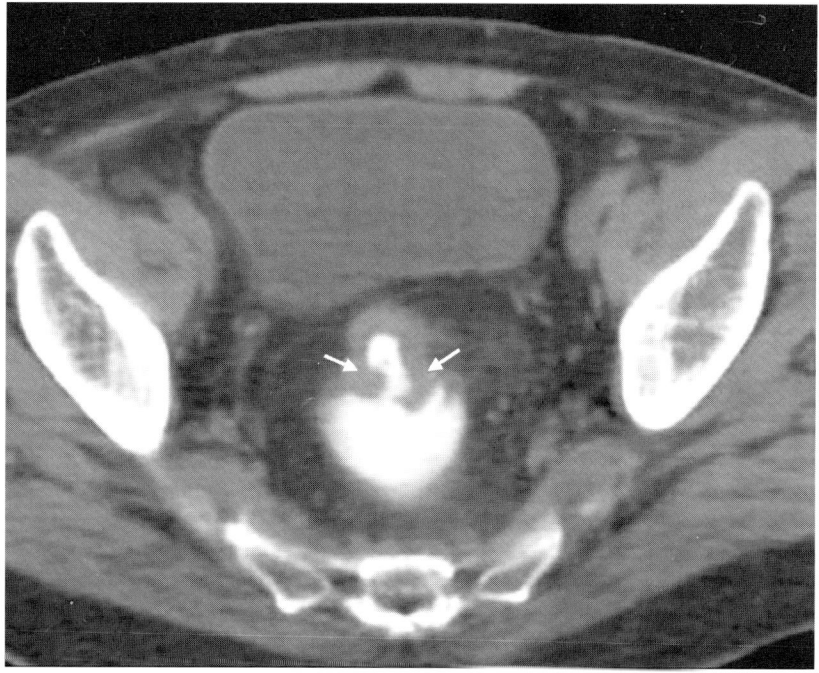

Fig. 1

Comments and Explanation

Colorectal carcinoma is common, accounting for 15% of all newly diagnosed cancers, and tends to be a disease of the elderly, with the median age of diagnosis between 60 and 80 years of age. Sigmoid colon is also involved in majority of cases. The tumor shows irregular walls and may show polypoidal growth or napkin ring growth pattern. Also it shows rapid spread to the surrounding in the form of fat stranding and destruction of fat planes. Colorectal cancers, 98% of which are adenocarcinomas, arise in majority of cases from pre-existing colonic adenomas (neoplastic polyps), which progressively undergo malignant transformation as they accumulate additional mutations.

Opinion

Sigmoid colon carcinoma.

Clinical Discussion

Clinical presentation is typically insidious, with altered bowel habit or iron deficiency anemia from chronic occult blood loss and non specific symptoms like fatigue and weight loss. Bowel obstruction, intussusception, heavy bleeding and metastatic disease may also be the initial manifestation. Colon cancer is now often detected during screening procedures. The incidence of colorectal cancer is about equal for males and females. Age is a well-known risk factor for colorectal cancer, as it is for many other solid tumors. The incidence of colorectal cancer peaks at about age 65 years. Other common clinical presentations include the following iron-deficiency anemia, rectal bleeding, abdominal pain, change in bowel habits, intestinal obstruction or perforation. CT scan findings associated with adenocarcinoma of colon include asymmetric bowel wall thickening with contrast enhancement or the presence of a soft-tissue mass that frequently leads to luminal narrowing or obstruction. Colorectal cancer may occasionally be associated with a wide spectrum of colonic complications that cause acute abdominal symptoms. Various complications such as obstruction, perforation, abscess formation, acute appendicitis, ischemic colitis and intussusception can occur in patients with colon cancer. Carcinomas of the transverse colon can spread via direct extension to stomach. Common sites of metastatic involvement include the liver, lungs, adrenal glands, peritoneum, and omentum. In females, the ovary may be involved. Surgery and chemotherapy are the mainstay of the treatment.

SECTION 8

Rectum

23. Carcinoma Rectum

CASE 23

Carcinoma Rectum

CASE

A 75-year-old male came with history of painless bleeding per rectum and weight loss was referred to the department of radiology for CT scan abdomen.

Radiological Findings on CT Examination

Axial post contrast CT images (Figs 1A and B) show ill defined, irregular, circumferential wall thickening of the rectum. The fat planes between rectal mass and rectovesical space is disturbed suggesting spread. The mass shows mild heterogeneous enhancement. Also there is evidence of involvement of few perirectal lymph nodes. These findings suggest rectal carcinoma with perirectal spread.

Axial post contrast CT images of another patient shows iso to hyperdense mass involving the lumen of the rectum. Also there are multiple hypodense lesions in both lobes of liver (Figs 1C and D). These findings suggest rectal carcinoma with hepatic metastases.

Comments and Explanation

Adenocarcinomas comprise the vast majority of colon and rectal cancers; more rare rectal cancers include lymphoma, carcinoid, and sarcoma. On CT these lesions are hypo to isodense with irregular margins and shows post contrast enhancement. The growth can be circumferential or intraluminal. Like colon cancer, rectal carcinoma also gives metastases to liver. Extrarectal tumor spread is suggested by a loss of tissue fat planes between the rectum and surrounding tissues, as well as perirectal fat stranding and nodularity. Invaded muscle may be enlarged. CT is used for staging rectal carcinomas before treatment, for staging of recurrent disease, and for detecting the presence of distant metastases after surgery. CT detects hepatic metastases as well-defined areas of low density in the portal venous phase, following injection of intravenous contrast medium. In the early arterial phase, hepatic metastases may demonstrate rim enhancement or become hyperdense or isodense in relation to normal liver.

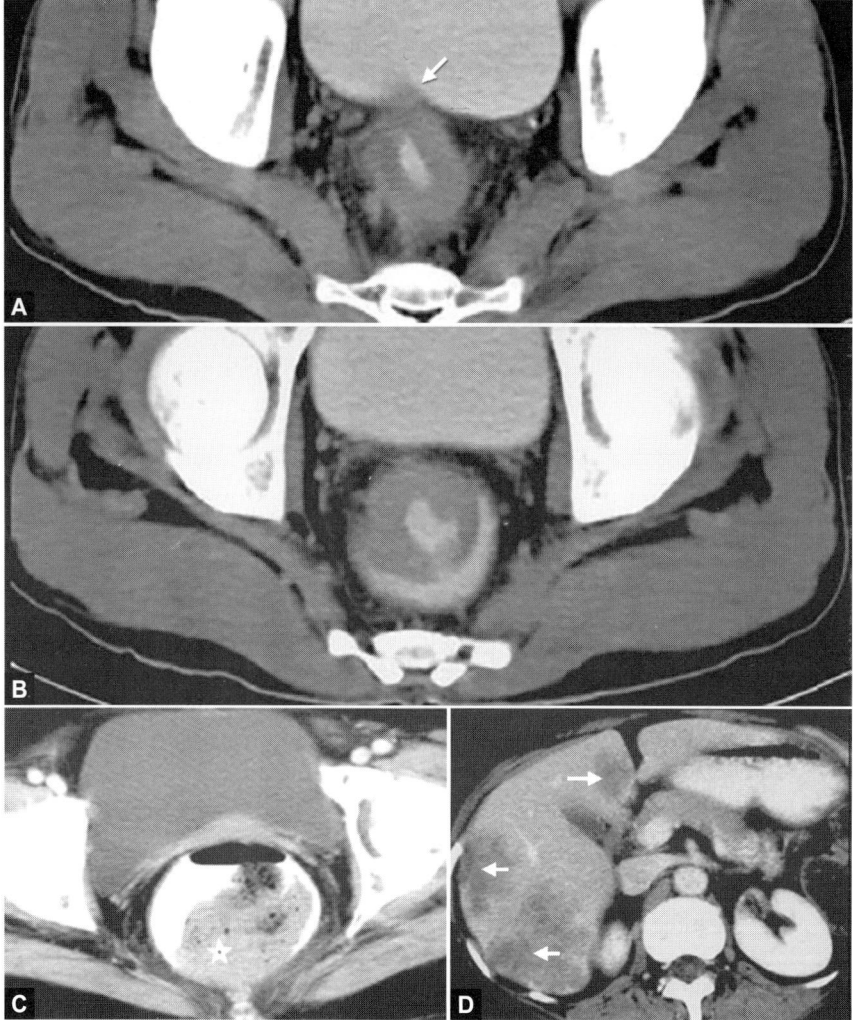

Figs 1A to D

Opinion

Rectal carcinoma.

Clinical Discussion

Rectal cancer is one of the most common tumor with a poor prognosis caused by high risk of local recurrence and metastasis. It is commonly seen in age group of 60 and above and has a male preponderance. Bleeding is the most common symptom of rectal cancer, occurring in 60% of patients. Occult bleeding is detected via a fecal occult blood test (FOBT) Abdominal pain is present in 20% of the cases. Partial large-bowel obstruction may cause colicky abdominal pain and bloating. Increased incidence of rectal carcinoma in western world is attributed to consumption of low fiber diet, red meat, and chronic constipation. The local recurrence is related to the extramural tumor spread into the mesorectum and to the tumor distance from circumferential resection margin (CRM). Imaging plays a crucial role in the preoperative management of rectal carcinoma because traditional techniques usually performed to make diagnosis (colonoscopy and digital rectal examination), do not adequately show important prognostic features such as depth of tumor spread T stage) or the extent of lymph node involvement (N stage). The mainstay of treatment is surgical excision; however pre-operative down-staging with either radiotherapy alone or combined chemo-radiotherapy is employed in T3 and/or N1 disease.

SECTION 9

Liver

24. Focal Fatty Liver
25. Simple Hepatic Cyst
26. Budd-Chiari Syndrome
27. Liver Laceration
28. Hepatic Abscess
29. Hepatic Hydatid Cyst
30. Hepatic Hemangioma
31. Focal Nodular Hyperplasia
32. Hepatic Adenoma
33. Hepatic Angiomyolipoma
34. Hepatocellular Carcinoma
35. Hepatic Metastases
36. Hepatoblastoma
37. Intrahepatic Cholangiocarcinoma
38. Extrahepatic Cholangiocarcinoma
39. Transient Hepatic Attenuation Difference

CASE 24

Focal Fatty Liver

CASE

A 52-year-old diabetic obese male was referred for CT abdomen as ultrasound was suggestive of a focal hyperechoic area in the liver. CT abdomen was done to rule out any focal liver lesion.

Radiological Findings on CT Scan

Non-enhanced CT (Fig. 1A) shows focal hypodense area in the liver. During the contrast phase of enhancement (Figs 1B to D) the intrahepatic vessels, i.e. the hepatic artery branches and portal vein follow the normal course in this hypodense area without distortion or mass effect. This area shows less enhancement than the rest of the liver on portal phase. This represent focal fatty infiltration of liver.

Comments and Explanation

Focal fatty liver (FFL) is localized or patchy process of lipid accumulation in the liver. It is likely to have different pathogenesis than nonalcoholic steatohepatitis which is a diffuse process. FFL may result from altered venous flow to liver, tissue hypoxia and malabsorption of lipoproteins. Focal fatty infiltration is distinguished on CT from space occupying lesions as focal fatty infiltration does not cause any mass effect or deformation of the organ. Typical location for focal fatty change is medial segment of the left lobe of the liver either anterior to the porta hepatis or adjacent to the falciform ligament. This distribution is the same as that seen in focal fatty sparing and is related to variations in vascular supply. On NECT it appears as a focal hypodense area which on CECT enhances less than the rest of the liver without distortion of intrahepatic vessels or mass effect.

Opinion

Focal fatty infiltration of liver.

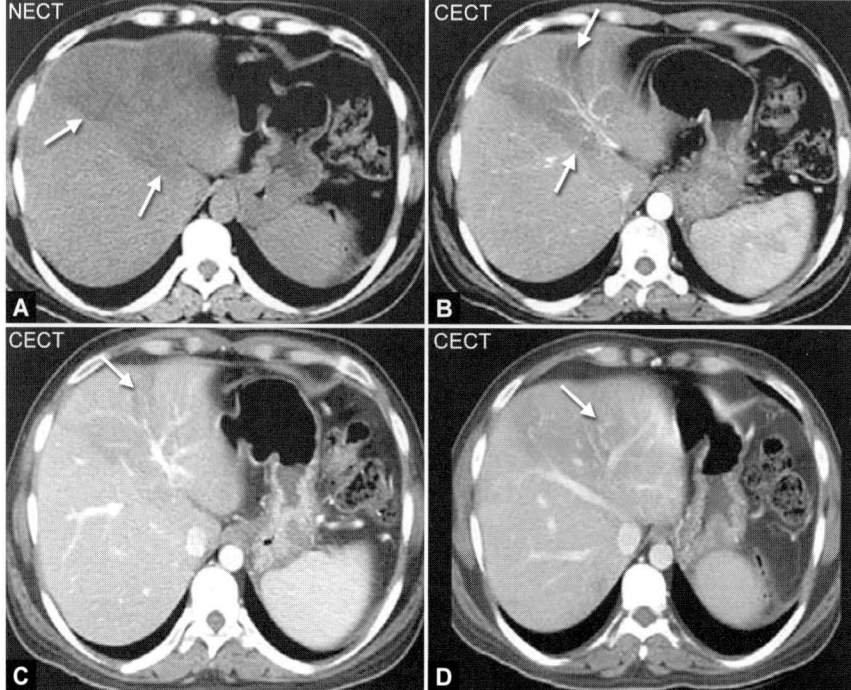

Figs 1A to D

Clinical Discussion

Focal fatty infiltration of liver is commonly seen in patients with diabetes mellitus, obesity, alcohol abuse, exogenous steroids, certain drugs, chemotherapy, and IV hyperalimentation.

Treatment of the underlying cause will reverse the findings. Liver with fatty change demonstrates increased echogenicity on ultrasound. The echogenic walls of the portal veins and hepatic veins are lost, due to the increased liver attenuation. MRI requires both in- and out-of-phase imaging and contrast to adequately assess. Pseudolesion (focal sparing) is better seen on out-of-phase imaging, but otherwise appears normal and similar to the rest of the liver on T2 and contrast enhanced sequences.

The diagnosis may be confirmed by biopsy and histopathology, however diagnosis of fat on CT and MR if often diagnostic and often needs no confirmation.

CASE 25

Simple Hepatic Cyst

CASE

A 40-year-old male presented to the department of radiology with dull pain in right hypochondriac region and was subjected to CT scan abdomen.

Radiological Findings on CT Examination

Axial plain (Fig. 1A) and post contrast (Fig. 1B) CT images of abdomen at the level of liver shows a large, well defined, thin walled, cystic lesion seen in right lobe of liver. The lesion shows smooth walls and there is no evidence of post contrast enhancement. There is no evidence of septae or calcification. Findings suggest simple hepatic cyst.

Comments and Explanation

Simple hepatic cyst is seen in 5% of the population. There is slight female predilection. These lesions may be isolated or multiple and vary from a few millimeters to several centimeters in diameter. Simple hepatic cysts are benign

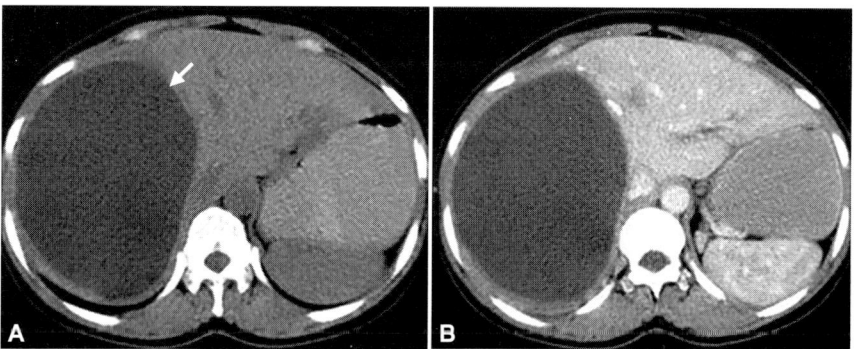

Figs 1A and B

developmental lesions that do not communicate with the biliary tree. They result from isolated aberrant biliary ducts. The cyst contents are usually clear serous fluid. They may cause obstruction or compression atrophy of the liver parenchyma when they attain a large size.

Few close differential diagnosis of simple cysts are as follows:
- *Benign developmental hepatic cyst:* It is benign, congenital, and developmental lesion which is derived from biliary endothelium that does not communicate with the biliary tree.
- *Von Meyenburg complex:* It is benign malformation of the biliary tract that originate from embryonic bile duct that fails to involute.
- Adult polycystic liver disease.

Opinion

Simple hepatic cyst.

Clinical Discussion

Simple hepatic cyst can occur anywhere in the liver, with greater predilection towards the right lobe of the liver. Simple cysts generally are asymptomatic but may produce dull right upper quadrant pain if large in size. Patients may present with abdominal bloating and early satiety. Occasionally, a large cyst is palpable as abdominal mass. Jaundice caused by bile duct obstruction is rare, as is cyst rupture and acute torsion of a mobile cyst. Patients with cyst torsion may present with an acute abdomen. When simple cysts rupture, patients may develop secondary infection, leading to a presentation similar to a hepatic abscess with abdominal pain, fever, and leukocytosis. The clinician has a number of options for imaging the liver in patients with hepatic cysts. Ultrasonography is readily available, noninvasive, and highly sensitive. Computed tomography scan is also highly sensitive and is easier for most clinicians to interpret, particularly for treatment planning. While planning for treatment of hepatic simple cysts, it needs to be differentiated from cystic neoplasm. Cystic neoplasms tend to have thicker, irregular, hypervascular walls, whereas simple cysts tend to be thin walled and uniform. Simple cysts tend to have homogenous low-density interiors, whereas neoplastic cysts usually have heterogeneous interiors with septa and papillary extrusions.

CASE 26

Budd-Chiari Syndrome

CASE

A 33-year-old female patient came to the radiology department with history of severe pain in abdomen and was subjected to CT abdomen.

Radiological Findings on CT Scan

Contrast enhanced CT abdomen (Figure 1) shows patchy nonenhancing hypodense areas in both lobes of liver, predominantly affecting the right lobe. There is nonvisualization of the right, middle and left hepatic veins. Portal vein, portal radicles, IVC appear normal. On the basis of these findings the diagnosis of Budd-Chiari syndrome needs to be considered.

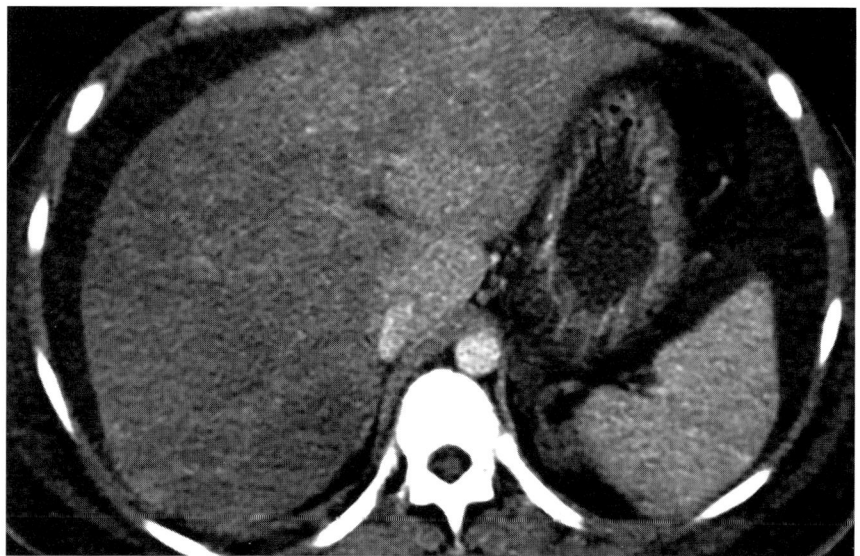

Fig. 1

Comments and Explanation

Budd-Chiari syndrome is a condition caused by occlusion of the hepatic veins that drain the liver. Caudate lobe hypertrophy is often present. Any obstruction of the venous vasculature of the liver is referred to as Budd-Chiari syndrome, from the venules to right atrium. This leads to increased portal vein and hepatic sinusoid pressures as the blood flow stagnates. The increased portal pressure causes increased filtration of vascular fluid with the formation of ascites in the abdomen and collateral venous flow through alternative veins leading to esophageal, gastric and rectal varices. Obstruction also causes centrilobular necrosis and peripheral lobule fatty change due to ischemia. If this condition persists chronically what is known as nutmeg liver will develop. Budd-Chiari syndrome is most commonly diagnosed using ultrasound studies of the abdomen and retrograde angiography. Ultrasound may show obliteration of hepatic veins, thrombosis or stenosis, spiderweb vessels, large collateral vessels, or a hyperechoic cord replacing a normal vein. Computed tomography (CT) or magnetic resonance imaging (MRI) is sometimes employed although these methods are generally not as sensitive. On CT there is inhomogeneous mottled liver with delayed enhancement in the periphery of the liver and around the hepatic veins (nutmeg liver), peripheral zones of the liver may appear hypoattenuating because of reversed portal venous blood flow caudate lobe enlargement and increased contrast enhancement compared with the remainder of the liver inability to identify hepatic veins.

Liver biopsy is nonspecific but sometimes necessary to differentiate between Budd-Chiari syndrome and other causes of hepatomegaly and ascites, such as galactosemia or Reye's syndrome.

Opinion

Budd-Chiari syndrome.

Clinical Discussion

It presents with the classical triad of abdominal pain, ascites and hepatomegaly. The syndrome can be acute, chronic, or asymptomatic. The acute syndrome presents with rapidly progressive severe upper abdominal pain, jaundice, hepatomegaly, ascites, elevated liver enzymes, and eventually encephalopathy. The fulminant syndrome presents early with encephalopathy and ascites. Severe hepatic necrosis and lactic acidosis may be present as well. Patients may progress to cirrhosis. It can be classified into primary and secondary types. (a) Primary Budd-Chiari syndrome (75%): thrombosis of the hepatic vein (b) Secondary Budd-Chiari syndrome (25%): compression of the hepatic vein by an outside structure (e.g. a tumor). Hepatic vein thrombosis is associated with pregnancy, postpartum state, use of oral contraceptives and hepatocellular carcinoma. Budd-Chiari syndrome is also seen in infections such as tuberculosis, congenital venous webs and occasionally in inferior vena caval stenosis. Often, the patient is known to have a tendency towards thrombosis, although Budd-Chiari syndrome can also be the first symptom of such a tendency. Examples of genetic tendencies include protein C deficiency, protein S deficiency, the Factor V Leiden mutation, hereditary anti-thrombin deficiency. An important nongenetic risk factor is the use of estrogen-containing (combined) forms of hormonal contraception. Other risk factors include the antiphospholipid syndrome, aspergillosis, Behçet's disease, dacarbazine, pregnancy, and trauma. Many patients have Budd-Chiari syndrome as a complication of polycythemia vera. Patients suffering from paroxysmal nocturnal hemoglobinuria (PNH) appear to be especially at risk for Budd-Chiari syndrome, more than other forms of thrombophilia: up to 39% develop venous thromboses and 12% may acquire Budd-Chiari.

CASE 27

Liver Laceration

CASE

A 43-year-old male came with history of trauma in a semiconscious state. CT abdomen was done to rule out injury to the abdominal organs.

Radiological Findings on CT Scan

CT findings show contusions and lacerations in the liver which are seen on CECT as irregular nonenhancing areas (Figs 1A and B). In case of severe trauma it can result in diaphragmatic rupture with herniation of liver in the thorax as shown in Figures 1C and D.

Comments and Explanation

The liver is the second most commonly injured organ in abdominal trauma, first being the spleen but damage to the liver is the most common cause of death after abdominal injury. Trauma to the liver may result in subcapsular or intrahepatic hematoma, contusion, vascular injury, or biliary disruption. The findings to look for in abdominal trauma are Hemoperitoneum, Contrast blush consistent with active extravasation, Laceration: linear shaped hypodense areas, Hematomas: oval or round shaped areas, Contusions: vague ill-defined hypodense areas that are less well perfused, pneumoperitoneum, devascularization of organs and subcapsular hematomas.

Opinion

Hepatic trauma.

Clinical Discussion

Contrast-enhanced CT is accurate in localizing the site and extent of liver injuries and associated trauma, providing vital information for treatment in patients. CT scans can be used to monitor healing. Trauma to the liver may

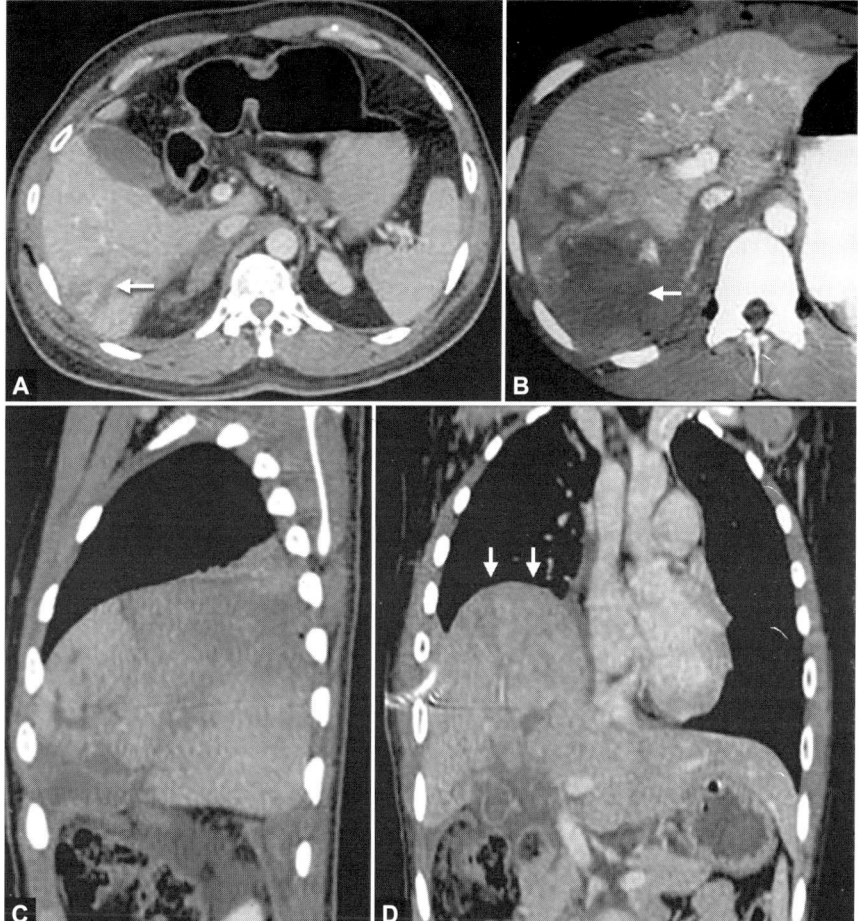

Figs 1A to D

result in subcapsular or intrahepatic hematoma, contusion, vascular injury, or biliary disruption. CT has made a great impact on the diagnosis of patients with liver trauma, and use of this technique has resulted in marked reduction in the number of patients requiring surgery. CT can also detect injury to other surrounding organs like pancreas, spleen, kidneys, etc.

CT criteria for the American Association of Surgery for Trauma (AAST) liver injury grading system for liver trauma is as follows:
- *Grade I:* Hematoma: sub capsular, <10% surface area, Laceration: capsular tear, < 1 cm depth.
- *Grade II:* Hematoma: sub capsular, 10–50% surface area, Hematoma: intraparenchymal <10 cm diameter, Laceration: capsular tear, 1–3 cm depth <10 cm length.
- *Grade III:* Hematoma: sub capsular, >50% surface area, or ruptured with active bleeding, Hematoma: intraparenchymal >10 cm diameter, Laceration: capsular tear, > 3 cm depth.

- *Grade IV:* Hematoma: ruptured intraparenchymal with active bleeding, Laceration: parenchymal disruption involving 25–75% hepatic lobes or involves 1–3 Couinaud segments (within one lobe).
- *Grade V:* Laceration: parenchymal distruption involving >75% hepatic lobe or involves > 3 Couinaud segments (within one lobe), Vascular: juxtahepatic venous injuries (IVC, major hepatic vein).
- *Grade VI:* Vascular: hepatic avulsion.

Pooling of contrast material within the peritoneal cavity indicates active and massive bleeding; patients with this finding may require emergency surgery. Intrahepatic pooling of contrast material with an intact liver capsule indicates a self-limiting hemorrhage. Vascular injury to the hepatic vein or IVC results when a laceration or contusion extends upto them with hemorrhage seen in the lesser sac or retrohepatic region. Pseudoaneurysms can be detected on dynamic angiographic studies. Biliary injury is rare and may result in biliary peritonitis.

CASE 28

Hepatic Abscess

CASE

A 45-year-old male patient came with history of fever with chills and pain in right hypochondrium since 5 days and was referred to radiology department for CT scan abdomen and pelvis.

Radiological findings on CT scan

Figure 1 shows multiple well defined irregularly marginated hypodense lesions of varying sizes in right lobe of liver. There is mild perilesional hypodensity in the liver parenchyma suggestive of edema.

In another case plain CT abdomen (Fig. 2A) shows a large well defined hypodense lesion with CT attenuation value 5–10 HU in the left lobe of liver. It shows a thick peripherally enhancing wall. There is mild perilesional edema (Fig. 2B).

Comments and Explanation

Hepatic abscesses are localized collections of necrotic inflammatory tissue caused by bacterial, parasitic or fungal agents. On ultrasound, large hepatic abscesses have an appearance ranging from hypoechoic to hyperechoic, with internal echoes and debris. Gas in hepatic abscesses causes high-intensity linear echoes with acoustic shadowing or reverberation artifacts. On CT, amebic abscesses usually appear as rounded, well-defined lesions with attenuation values that indicate the presence of complex fluid (10–20 HU). An enhancing wall and a peripheral zone of edema around the abscess are common characteristic for this lesion. The central abscess cavity may show multiple septa, fluid-debris levels and rarely, air bubbles. Pyogenic abscesses are usually multiple and may be caused by hematogenous dissemination (of either gastrointestinal infection via the portal vein or disseminated sepsis via the hepatic artery), ascending cholangitis, or superinfection of necrotic tissue. Pyogenic abscesses may be classified as either microabscesses (<2 cm) or macroabscesses (>2 cm). Pyogenic micro abscesses may appear as multiple widely scattered lesions or as a cluster

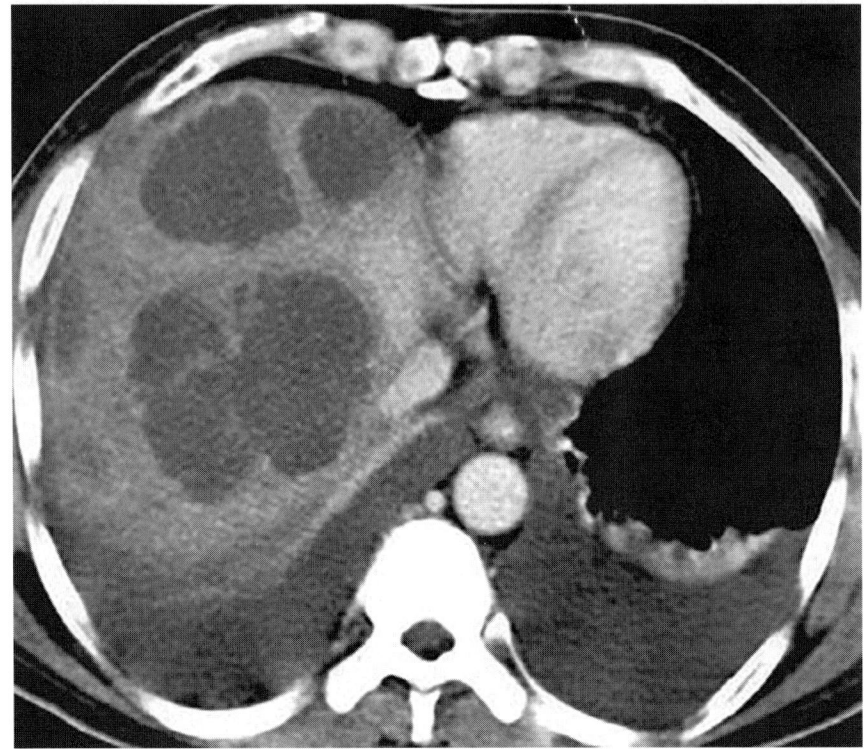

Fig. 1

of microabscesses that appear to coalesce focally (Cluster sign). It is likely that clustering of pyogenic microabscesses represents an early stage in the evolution of a large pyogenic abscess cavity. On contrast enhanced CT they appear as multiple small, well-defined hypoattenuating lesions with rim enhancement and perilesional edema. On contrast-enhanced CT, large abscesses are generally unilocular well defined and hypoattenuating with smooth margins or complex with internal septa and irregular margins. During arterial phase a double target sign is seen, the area around the center which is not enhanced is stained while the outermost layer shows hypodensity. In the portal to equilibrium phase a thick ring like stain is seen owing to staining of the outermost layers. Fungal abscess is caused by an opportunistic infection in immunocompromised patients. It presents as microabscesses which show faint ring like enhancement in arterial phase and hypodensity in the equilibrium phase.

Opinion

Hepatic abscess.

Case 28: Hepatic Abscess

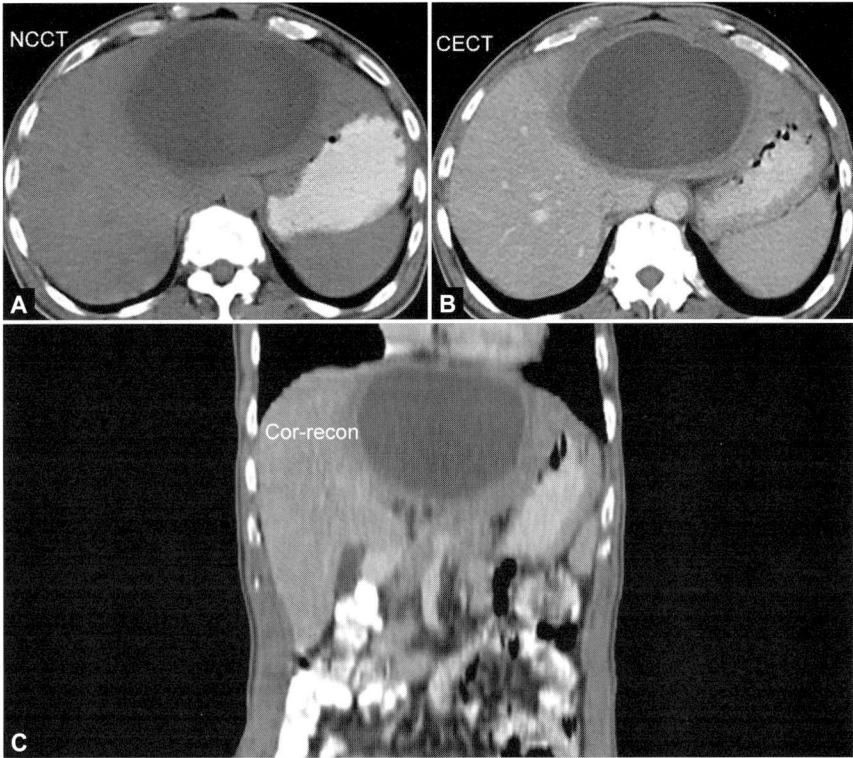

Figs 2A to C

Clinical Discussion

The typical presentation is right upper quadrant pain, fever and jaundice. Amebic liver abscess is the most common extraintestinal complication of amebiasis and commonly seen in a sub-diaphragmatic location and are likely to spread through the diaphragm into the chest. As a general rule, bacterial and fungal abscesses are often multiple, whereas amoebic abscesses are more frequently single. The presentation of liver abscess is dependent on the way the bacteria have entered the liver. Bacteria gets into the liver by four routes. The common route is through the portal vein. As a result of abdominal infection the bacteria enter through the slow flow portal system and they are layered within the vessel. In sepsis the spread is via the arterial system as in patients with endocarditis and there are multiple abscesses spread out through the periphery of the liver.

CASE 29

Hepatic Hydatid Cyst

CASE

A 56-year-old male patient with pain in abdomen was referred to radiology department for CT scan.

Radiological Findings on CT Scan

Plain CT scan abdomen (Fig. 1A) shows a well defined cystic lesion in left lobe of liver. Multiple small peripherally arranged cysts are seen within this lesion, these represent daughter cysts. There is no calcification or solid component within this lesion. Contrast enhanced CT scan shows cyst wall enhancement (Fig. 1B).

Comments and Explanation

Hydatid cysts result from infection by the echinococcus worm, and can result in cyst formation anywhere in the body. The ultrasonographic appearance of hydatid cysts may vary. The cyst wall usually manifests as double echogenic lines separated by a hypoechogenic layer. Multiple echogenic foci due to hydatid sand may be seen. The cyst may appear as a well-defined fluid collection with a

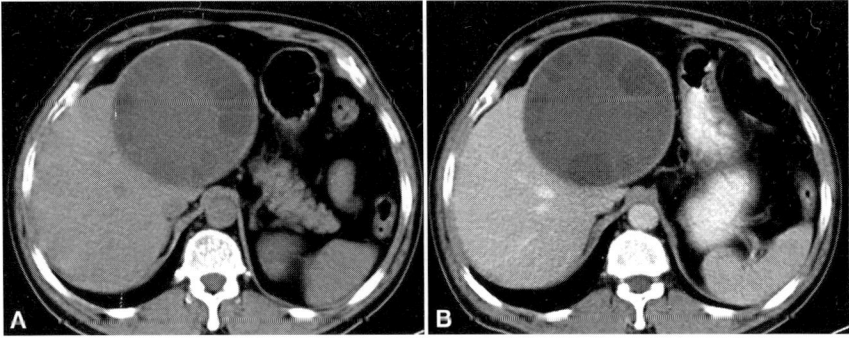

Figs 1A and B

localized split in the wall and "floating membranes" inside the cavity. Complete detachment of the membranes inside the cyst has been referred to as the ultrasound water lily sign. USG is the most sensitive modality for the detection of membranes, septa, and hydatid sand within the cyst. Multivesicular cysts manifest as well-defined fluid collections in a honeycomb pattern with multiple septa representing the walls of the daughter cysts. Daughter cysts appear as cysts within a cyst. Cyst calcification usually occurs in the cyst wall. When the cyst wall is heavily calcified, only the anterior portion of the wall is visualized and appears as a thick arch with a posterior concavity. CT may display the same findings as USG. Cyst usually demonstrates fluid attenuation (3–30 HU). Calcification of the cyst wall or internal septa is easily detected at CT. A hydatid cyst typically demonstrates a high-attenuation wall at unenhanced CT even without calcification. Detachment of the laminated membrane from the pericyst can be visualized as linear areas of increased attenuation within the cyst. Daughter cysts manifest as round structures located peripherally within the mother cyst. Intrahepatic complications of hydatid cysts include cyst rupture and infection. Cyst rupture results in free spillage of hydatid material into the peritoneal cavity, pleural cavity, hollow viscera, abdominal wall, and so on. Both USG and CT may demonstrate a cyst wall defect and passage of the cyst contents through the defect in direct communication. Infection occurs only after rupture of both the pericyst and endocyst which allows bacteria to pass easily into the cyst. CT is the modality of choice for demonstrating cyst infection. Infected cysts may manifest at CT as poorly defined masses, in contrast to the more clearly defined masses seen in uncomplicated cases. Contrast-enhanced CT may reveal the typical high-attenuation rim representing abscesses surrounding the lesion. CT clearly depicts gas or air-fluid levels within the cyst. Involvement of the diaphragm and thoracic cavity occurs in 0.6%–16% of cases of hepatic hydatid disease. Transdiaphragmatic migration varies from simple adherence to the diaphragm to rupture into the pleural cavity, seeding in the pulmonary parenchyma, and chronic bronchial fistula. Peritoneal echinococcosis is almost always secondary to hepatic disease. CT is the modality of choice in such cases as it allows imaging of the entire abdomen and pelvis. Cysts may be multiple and located anywhere in the peritoneal cavity.

Opinion

Hepatic hydatid cyst.

Clinical Discussion

Hepatic hydatid disease is a parasitic zoonosis caused by the echinococcus tape worm. In the liver, two agents are recognized as causing disease in the human: echinococcus granulosus and echinococcus alveolaris. Hydatid cyst consists of 3 layers—endocyst (single layer lining the inner aspect of the cyst), ectocyst (middle layer easily separable from the adventitia) and pericyst (outer adventitia). Daughter vesicles (brood capsules) are small spheres that contain the protoscolices and are formed from rests of the germinal layer. Before becoming daughter cysts, these daughter vesicles are attached by a pedicle to the germinal layer of the mother cyst. Hydatid cysts are slow growing at the rate of

1–1.5 cm per year. Once the parasite passes through the intestinal wall to reach the portal venous system or lymphatic system, the liver acts as the first line of defense and is therefore the most frequently involved organ. The right lobe is the most frequently involved portion of the liver. CT scanning has the advantage of inspecting any organ, detecting smaller cysts when located outside the liver. MRI may have some advantages over CT scanning in the evaluation of postsurgical residual lesions, recurrences, and selected extrahepatic infections, such as cardiac infections. It is also superior in identifying changes of the intrahepatic and extrahepatic venous system and in identifying cysto-biliary fistulas.

CASE

30 Hepatic Hemangioma

CASE

A 50-year-old patient came with history of pain in abdomen and vomiting and was referred to radiology department for CT scan.

Radiological Findings on CT Examination

Plain CT abdomen (Fig. 1A) shows a well defined hyperdense lesion in segment IV of left lobe of liver. CT in arterial phase (Fig. 1B) shows peripheral discontinuous nodular enhancement. Portal phase (Fig. 1C) and delayed image (Fig. 1D) show gradual centripetal filling of the lesion. This lesion represents hemangioma.

Comments and Explanation

It is the most common benign hepatic tumor in clinical practice. It is seen in all age groups and has a female preponderance. It is detected in the absence of signs and symptoms in almost all cases. They are lined by a single layer of endothelial cells and are composed of large vascular channels filled with slowly moving blood. When the tumor exceeds 4 cm, abdominal pain or discomfort or a palpable mass may be present. Rupture occurs rarely. Hemangiomas are usually solitary but are multiple in approximately 10% of cases. Their borders are clear, but they are not encapsulated. As the hemangioma grows, various degenerative changes are seen in its center, including old and new thrombus formation, necrosis, scarring, hemorrhage, and calcification. When degeneration and fibrous changes become more prominent, the lesion is referred to as a sclerosed hemangioma.

Opinion

Hepatic hemangioma.

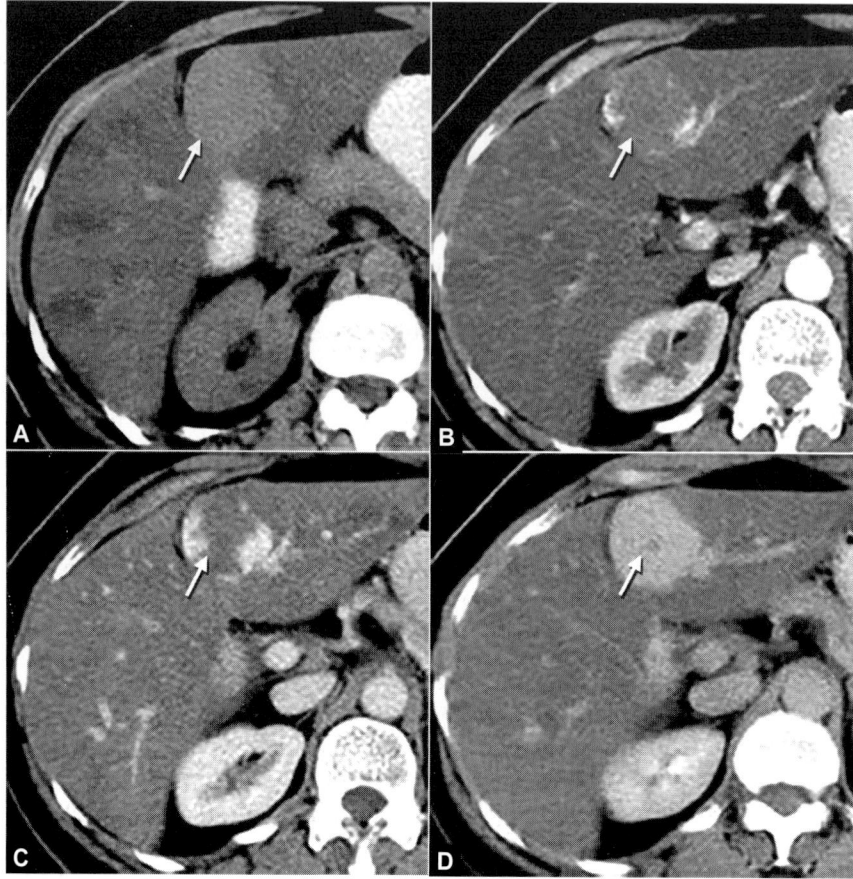

Figs 1A to D

Clinical Discussion

Hemangioma occurs more commonly in women. These lesions tend to be stable, but may enlarge during pregnancy or with estrogen administration. Hemangiomas are usually asymptomatic and are discovered incidentally. Large lesions can cause pain, nausea, or vomiting secondary to extrinsic compression of adjacent bowel, rupture, hemorrhage, or thrombosis. On ultrasound they are usually homogeneous well-defined hyperechoic masses with posterior acoustic enhancement. In the background of fatty liver hemangiomas may appear hypoechoic. Giant lesions can appear heterogeneous due to internal complex composition. Calcification is rare and is seen usually in the central scar of a giant hemangioma. On nonenhanced CT, hemangioma is depicted as a well-demarcated hypodense lesion. It is sometimes round but more often oval or irregular. Large lesions sometimes have a geographic (irregular) shape. In the arterial phase of dynamic CT, peripheral discontinuous nodular enhancement is seen first, followed by gradual filling toward the center (centripetal filling) and prolonged enhancement on the equilibrium phase—a pattern characteristic of hemangioma. The density of hemangiomas reflects the vascular spaces, and on precontrast, arterial and equilibrium phase dynamic CT, the fact that the tumor's density is similar to that of the aorta is useful diagnostic proof. In small hemangioma containing small sinusoids, dynamic CT may show the entire tumor to be enhanced from the early phase. The differential includes hypervascular metastases but these wash out on delayed imaging, and remain hypodense to the normal hepatic parenchyma whereas hemangiomas remain hyperdense on delayed images. Large hemangiomas can have an atypical appearance. Complete fill in is prevented in giant hemangiomas owing to central fibrous scarring. Calcification and cystic degeneration are also found in some cases. These lesions need to be differentiated from other lesions with a scar like fibrolamellar carcinoma, focal nodular hyperplasia, and cholangiocarcinoma.

CASE 31

Focal Nodular Hyperplasia

CASE

A 45-year-old woman with complaint of pain in right hypochondriac region came for CT abdomen and pelvis.

Radiological Findings on CT Examination

Plain CT (Fig. 1A) shows isodense solid mass in liver with hypodense central scar. On arterial phase (Fig. 1B) the lesion shows mild heterogeneous enhancement. On portal and venous phases (Figs 1C and D) the hypodense central scar

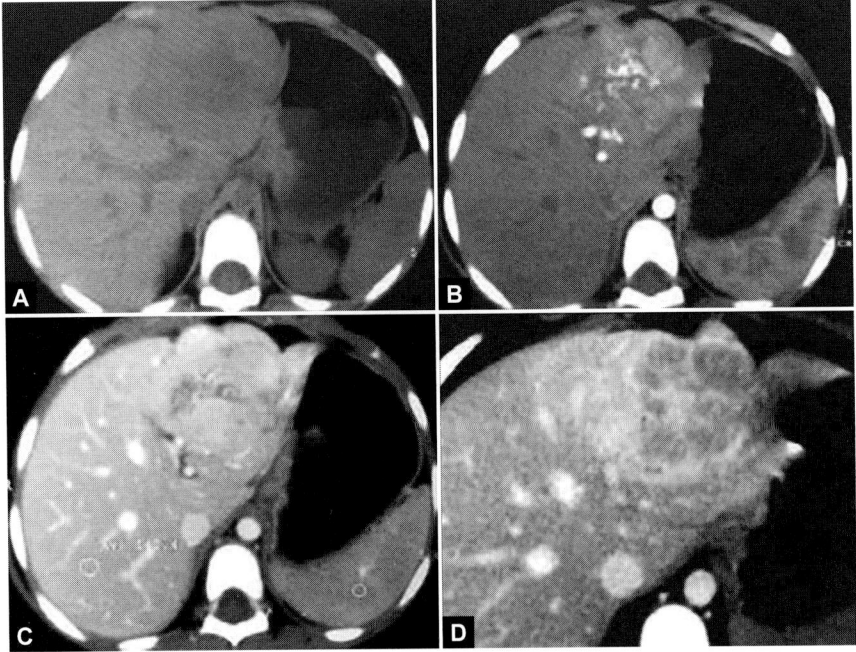

Figs 1A to D

shows enhancement. This turned out to be focal nodular hyperplasia on histopathological examination.

Comments and Explanation

Focal nodular hyperplasia is benign lesion and does not require treatment unless causing mass effect or pain. On ultrasound the lesions may be hypoechoic, isoechoic, or slightly hyperechoic. Some lesions may show a hypoechoic halo surrounding the lesion. This halo most likely represents compressed hepatic parenchyma or vessels surrounding the lesion. Currently, multirow detector CT does allow triphasic or even multiphasic dynamic contrast material–enhanced imaging in relatively shorter scanning times. Typical FNH may have lobulated contours on CT. On unenhanced CT, the lesions are either hypoattenuating or isoattenuating to the surrounding liver. In the arterial phase, the lesions become hyperattenuating due to the homogeneous intense enhancement of the entire lesion, except the central scar. In the portal and later phases, the lesions become more isoattenuating with the surrounding liver and the central scar may show some enhancement. The delayed enhancement of the central scar at CT and MR imaging relates to increased interstitial space and fluid content with slow diffusion of contrast material into this space.

Opinion

Focal nodular hyperplasia.

Clinical Discussion

Focal nodular hyperplasia (FNH) is the second most common tumor of the liver, after hepatic hemangioma. It is a benign hepatic tumor that likely represents a local hyperplastic response of hepatocytes to a congenital arteriovenous malformation. Though the use of contraceptives has not been implicated in the pathogenesis of FNH, their use is associated with the risk of complications with FNH. Use of contraceptives may be a factor in the development of FNH. In symptomatic females, hemorrhagic foci or infarctions may occur within the FNH. The rare complication is spontaneous rupture into the peritoneum. Most patients are asymptomatic, and FNH is incidentally discovered during cross-sectional imaging, angiography, radionuclide liver scanning, or surgery. In most cases, FNH occurs as a solitary lesion (80–95%) measuring less than 5 cm in diameter, but multiple lesions may occur. Although FNH usually has no clinical significance, recognition of the radiologic characteristics of FNH is important to avoid unnecessary surgery, biopsy, and follow-up imaging. Malignant transformation of FNH has not been observed.

CASE 32

Hepatic Adenoma

CASE

A 40-year-old female patient came with complaints of pain in right hypochondriac region and was referred to radiology department for CT scan.

Radiological Findings on CT Examination

Plain CT (Fig. 1A) shows hyperdense mass in right lobe of liver. There is homogeneous enhancement in the post contrast image (Fig. 1B) returning to near isodensity on portal venous and delayed phase image (not shown in image).

Comments and Explanation

The majority of hepatic adenomas contain fat and glycogen. In most cases, nonenhanced CT depicts this tumor as a hypodense mass. Small tumors appear

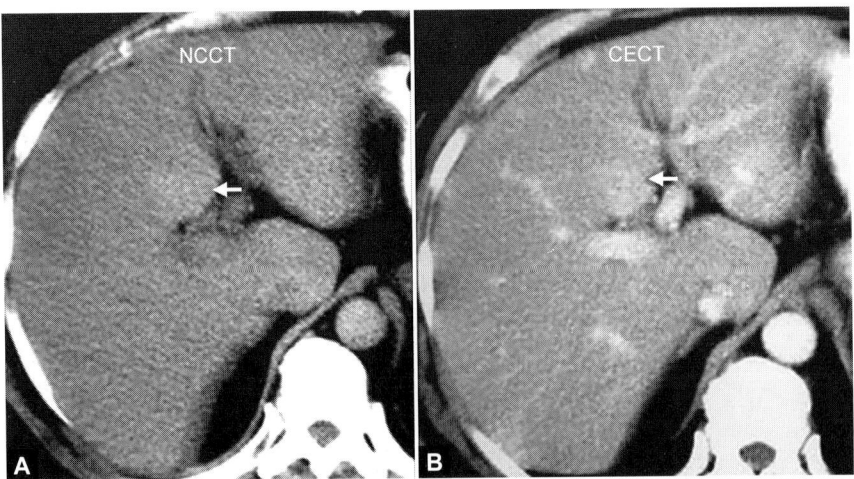

Figs 1A and B

homogeneous, but in general, the center shows inhomogeneous attenuation. Coagulum or thrombus may be noted in relatively early stages of ruptured hepatic adenoma as areas of hyperattenuation. In tumors with marked fatty metamorphosis of hepatocytes, a fat-related hypodense area may be seen. In addition, necrotic foci and scar tissue may appear as hypodense areas. Calcification is seen within the tumor in some cases. In the arterial phase of dynamic CT, moderate tumor enhancement is seen. In general they are well marginated and iso attenuating to liver. On contrast administration they demonstrate transient relatively homogeneous enhancement returning to near isodensity on portal venous and delayed phase image. Unfortunately, this homogeneous enhancement in the late arterial phase is not specific to adenomas, since small HCC's, hemangiomas as well as hypervascular metastases and FNH can demonstrate similar enhancement in the arterial phase. Malignant lesions however have a tendency to loose their contrast faster than the surrounding liver, so they may become relatively hypodense in later phases. The pathologic and the imaging differentiation between hepatic adenoma and well-differentiated HCC are not simple. Significant overlap is noted between the CT appearances of adenoma, HCC, FNH, and hypervascular metastases, making a definitive diagnosis based on CT imaging criteria alone difficult and often not possible. Clinical correlation in such cases is most helpful. In otherwise healthy young women using oral contraceptives, adenoma is favored.

Opinion

Hepatic adenoma.

Clinical Discussion

A hepatic adenoma is an uncommon benign liver tumor that is hormone induced. It tends to occur in young women compared to FNH and most of whom have a history of oral contraceptive use. Patients with hepatic adenoma usually present with an abdominal mass or recurrent abdominal pain, but the presentation can also present as acute abdomen owing to tumor rupture. In this case, the patient may develop shock because of intraperitoneal bleeding. Hepatic adenoma develops in noncirrhotic livers and is usually solitary but may occur in multiple forms. Lesions protruding from the liver surface are common, with pedunculated growth. The tumor border is clear and there is usually no capsule, although part of the tumor or its entire circumference may be covered by a fibrous capsule in some cases. In its core, bleeding, necrosis, and scar tissue are seen. They typically measure 8-15 cm and consist of sheets of well-differentiated hepatocytes. Adenomas are prone to central necrosis and hemorrhage because the vascular supply is limited to the surface of the tumor. There is also association of the tumor and glycogen storage disease. There is a very small risk of transformation to hepatocellular carcinoma. In general adenomas are resected, both to eliminate the risk of spontaneous rupture and to confirm the diagnosis. In inoperable cases, hepatic arterial embolization may have a role.

CASE 33

Hepatic Angiomyolipoma

CASE

A 50-year-old male patient with pain in right side of abdomen was referred to radiology department for CT scan abdomen.

Radiological Findings on CT Examination

Plain CT abdomen (Fig. 1A) shows a well defined hypodense heterogeneous lesion in right lobe of liver. It has small amount of fatty component. Contrast enhanced CT scan (Fig. 1B) shows multiple enhancing vessels within this lesion. Ultrasound (Fig. 1C) shows a well defined lobulated homogenously hyperechoic lesion in right lobe of liver. These findings are suggestive of angiomyolipoma.

Comments and Explanation

Angiomyolipoma (AML) is an uncommon benign hepatic mass lesion, containing blood vessel (angioid), smooth muscle (myoid) and mature fat (lipoid) components. The characteristic findings on any modality are the presence of both fat and prominent vascularity in the same lesion. If the fatty component predominates, it resembles lipomas but most of the time, a mixture of usual solid soft tissue and fatty components will be seen. The drainage vein of AML is the hepatic vein, and identifying a perfusing vein communicating with hepatic vein from the tumor center can aid in differentiating AML from fat containing hepatocellular carcinoma. On USG it appears hetero or homogeneous echogenic (due to fat content) mass lesion in right hepatic lobe and could be indistinguishable from hemangioma. Color Doppler sonography shows punctiform or filiform vascular distribution pattern if the tumor has predominance of angiomatous tissue. On nonenhanced CT, angiomyolipoma presents as well defined solid heterogeneous mass containing hypodense areas. Due to presence of the vascular component, marked enhancement in arterial phase is evident. Drainage is via the hepatic veins and this is the main differentiating point from fat containing hepatocellular carcinoma (HCC) that drains mainly in portal vein. It shows significant enhancement in arterial phase. On portal phase the lesion becomes hypoattenuated. Hypervascularity and tumor stain is seen on angiography.

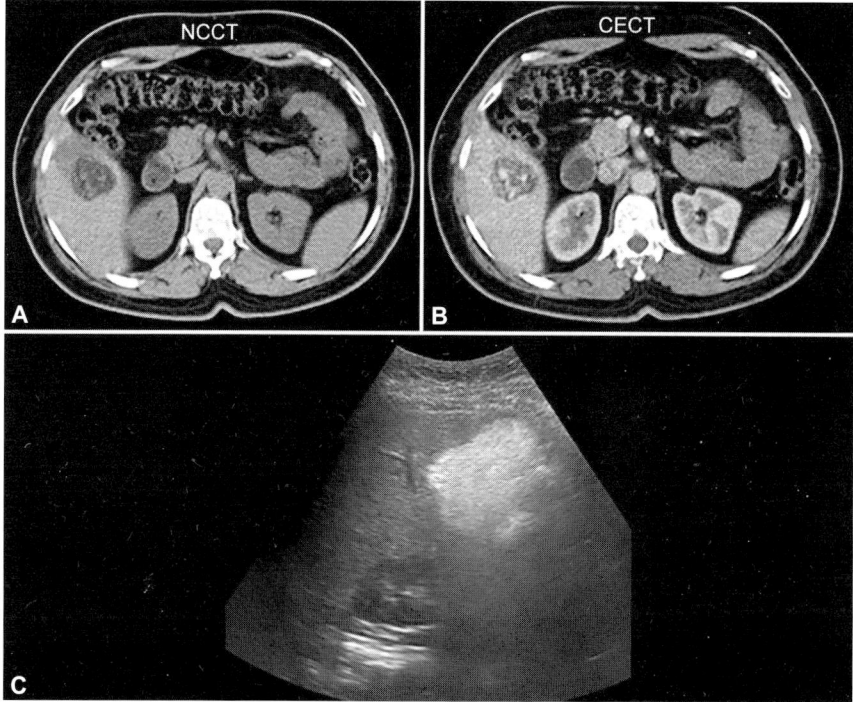

Figs 1A to C

Opinion

Hepatic angiomyolipomas.

Clinical Discussion

Most cases of angiomyolipoma are detected incidentally. Angiomyolipomas may be single or multiple, round or lobulated fat containing mass lesions, seen more commonly in the right lobe of liver. AMLs are usually found in the kidneys in patients with tuberous sclerosis. Multiple hepatic AMLs associated with renal AMLs should raise the suspicion for tuberous sclerosis. AMLs can be difficult to diagnose on imaging studies as the proportion of vessels, muscle and fatty tissue vary. Since hepatic AMLs usually follow benign clinical courses, the majority of the cases can be conservatively treated. Careful follow-up of the tumor even after the final diagnosis is necessary. We propose that tumor resection is indicated in the following scenarios: (1) the patients show symptoms; (2) the tumor shows an aggressive growth; (3) the tumor shows invasive growth into the vessels evidenced by fine-needle biopsy or imaging studies; (4) the component of the tumor shows atypical epithelioid pattern, high proliferation activity, and/or p53 immunoreactivity; and (5) a definitive diagnosis cannot be made by imaging and pathological studies from malignant tumors.

CASE 34

Hepatocellular Carcinoma

CASE

A 60-year-old male with right upper quadrant pain was referred to radiology department for CT scan.

Radiological Findings on CT Examination

In Figure 1(A) plain CT abdomen shows mass in liver; (B) Arterial phase CT shows enhancement in the mass. A hypodense scar is also seen (arrow); (C) Venous phase CT shows enhancement in the mass as well as the scar (arrow); (D) In delayed phase CT there is persistence of contrast in the scar. This differentiates it from fibronodular hyperplasia.

Comments and Explanation

Hepatocellular carcinoma (HCC) is the most common malignancy of liver. The CT appearance of HCC is variable and depends not only on the size, vascularity, histologic composition, and growth pattern of the tumor, but on the CT technique used, most HCCs are hypoattenuating on precontrast images, but a significant minority is isoattenuating to liver parenchyma prior to IV contrast medium administration. Some of the isoattenuating lesions can be identified on unenhanced images by the presence of a hypoattenuating rim, which represents the tumor capsule, or by a focal bulge in the contour of the liver. On rare occasions, the mass may extend exophytically beyond the confines of the liver and stimulate an extra hepatic mass. Areas of necrosis or fatty metamorphosis appear as hypoattenuating foci within the mass, whereas recent hemorrhage may produce areas of hyper attenuation. Calcification is identified in approximately 5-10% of HCCs. Precontrast images are important to identify lesions that are hyper attenuating prior to contrast medium administration (e.g. from hemorrhage or iron deposition) to avoid mistaking the increased attenuation on post contrast images as lesion enhancement. On delayed images, areas of fibrosis, including the capsule and septa, usually demonstrate prolonged enhancement. Diffusely infiltrating HCCs are best seen during the late hepatic

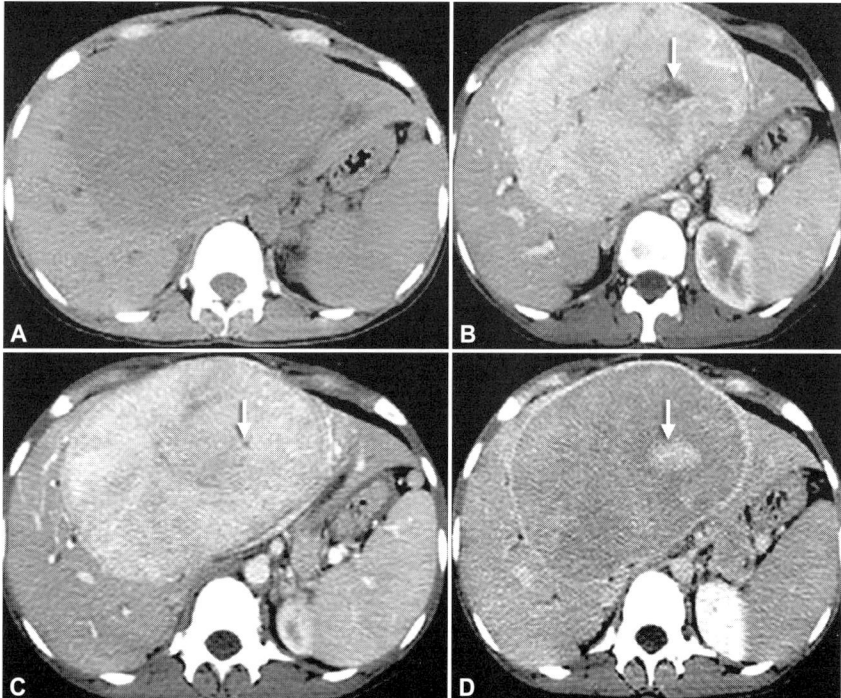

Figs 1A to D

arterial phase as ill-defined, vaguely nodular areas of hyper attenuation without discrete margins, but such lesions may be difficult to detect during any phase of enhancement. Contrast-enhanced CT is capable of demonstrating both vascular invasion and arterioportal shunting associated with HCC. Portal or hepatic vein tumor thrombus appears as a hypoattenuating filling defect within the expanded vascular lumen. Intravascular tumor thrombus may show homogeneous or streaky contrast enhancement, distinguishing it from bland thrombus. Signs of arterioportal shunting include early or prolonged enhancement of the portal vein and transient segmental, lobar or wedge-shaped hyper enhancement peripheral to the tumor. Hepatocellular carcinoma may cause biliary ductal dilation by compressive effect or, less commonly, by direct ductal invasion. Lesions that occur in noncirrhotic livers tend to be larger and are more frequently solitary than those occurring in cirrhotic livers.

Opinion

Hepatocellular carcinoma.

Clinical Discussion

Hepatocellular carcinoma is the fifth most common cancer in the world. The various risk factors associated are infection with hepatitis virus infection

Hepatitis C, B, alcoholism and aflatoxin ingestion. The gross features of HCC are classified into five major types: (1) small nodular with indistinct margin; (2) simple nodular; (3) simple nodular with extra nodular growth; (4) confluent multinodular; and (5) infiltrative. Patients with small, localized tumors usually have no HCC-related symptoms. In the advanced terminal stage patients, upper abdominal mass, abdominal pain, general malaise, anorexia, abdominal fullness, weight loss, jaundice, ascites, edema, and gastrointestinal bleeding are commonly present. The macro nodular cirrhosis is most often associated with HCC rather than micro nodular HCC. Intraperitoneal bleeding (rupture) is one of the most serious complications of advanced tumors, although it may occur in smaller lesions as well. Most HCCs develop in cirrhotic livers. Therefore, it has become possible to detect small, early-stage HCC in these high-risk patients. If the lesion is small then resection is possible (partial hepatectomy) and may result in cure. Liver transplantation is also a curative option.

CASE

35

Hepatic Metastases

CASE

A 60-year-old male, known case of mucinous carcinoma of transverse colon came for CT abdomen and pelvis.

Radiological Findings on CT Examination

Figure 1A contrast CT abdomen shows differential enhancement in the left lobe and an ill-defined low density mass which was hepatic metastases from mucinous carcinoma of transverse colon. Enlarged liver shows multiple round hypodense metastatic lesions in both the lobes (Figs 1B to D). Those of which are more hypodense in center indicate onset of necrosis.

Comments and Explanation

CT is the study of choice for evaluating liver metastases. On ultrasound, hepatic metastases appear as well defined rounded hypoechoic lesions. Cystic, calcified, infiltrative and echogenic appearances are all possible. In bull's eye, or target metastases, the halo is most probably related to a combination of compressed normal hepatic parenchyma around the mass and a zone of cancer cell proliferation. Most liver metastases are hypovascular compared with surrounding parenchyma and therefore most lesions appear either hypoattenuating or isoattenuating relative to the surrounding normal liver on unenhanced CT. Hypovascular lesions are more easily detected using contrast-enhancement. On contrast-enhanced scans, liver metastases may display slight peripheral enhancement with a hypoattenuating center. The margin of the lesions can vary from well defined to ill defined. Hyperattenuating lesions are uncommon. On the portal venous phase of scanning, some highly vascular primary tumors such as renal cell carcinomas, pancreatic islet cell tumors, pheochromocytomas, melanomas, and breast carcinomas, may appear as isoattenuating to normal liver. Differential diagnosis include, multiple hemangiomas which can be mistaken for metastases, focal nodular hyperplasia (FNH) may look like vascular metastases.

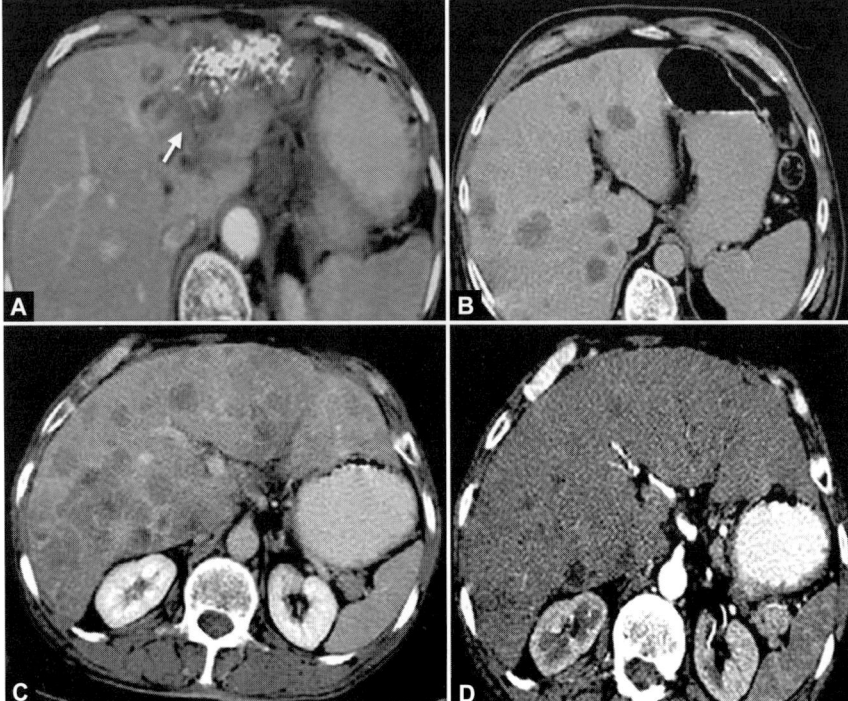

Figs 1A to D

Focal fatty sparing in a diffusely fatty liver can also look like metastases. MRI is usually used as problem-solving rather than a primary technique in the diagnosis of liver metastases. Most liver tumors, benign or malignant, appear as hypo intense lesions on T1-weighted images and hyper intense lesions on T2-weighted images. Gadolinium-enhanced MRI improves both the detection of focal liver masses and the differentiation of benign from malignant lesions. Multiple hepatic nodules of different sizes within the liver are nearly always due to metastases.

Opinion

Hepatic metastases.

Clinical Discussion

Metastasis is the most common neoplasm in an adult liver. The liver is a principle target for gastrointestinal malignancies. The most common primary sites for metastatic lesions to the liver in adults are colon, stomach, pancreas, breast, lung, and eye. In children, most common primary sites for metastatic lesions to the liver are neuroblastoma, Wilms' tumor, and leukemia. Most liver metastases are multiple. Multiple lesions often vary in size suggesting tumor seeding which occurs episodically. About half of patients with liver metastases have clinical signs of hepatomegaly or ascites. Liver function tests tend to be insensitive and nonspecific. Almost all tumors that metastasize to the liver also metastasize elsewhere at the same time. Some tumors, such as colon carcinoma, carcinoid, and hepatocellular carcinoma (HCC) may present with lesions confined to the liver. The pathology of metastatic deposits in the liver closely resembles the primary tumor, i.e. they are usually as vascular as their primary tumors. In general, most metastases are hypovascular, but some primaries characteristically have hypervascular metastases. The most common primary for hypervascular metastases are carcinoids, leiomyosarcomas, neuroendocrine tumors, renal carcinomas, thyroid carcinomas, choriocarcinomas occasionally pancreas, ovary, or breast carcinomas. Blood flow increases in all metastases, even hypovascular tumors. Neovascularity, vascular encasement, and arteriovenous shunting are rare. Large metastases can outgrow their blood supply leading to central necrosis.

CASE 36

Hepatoblastoma

CASE

A 12-year-old male child with history of anorexia, vomiting and jaundice was referred to the department of radiology for CT abdomen and pelvis.

Radiological Findings on CT Examination

Figure 1 contrast enhanced CT scan abdomen is showing heterogeneous large mass involving left lobe of liver with areas of necrosis and hemorrhage. There

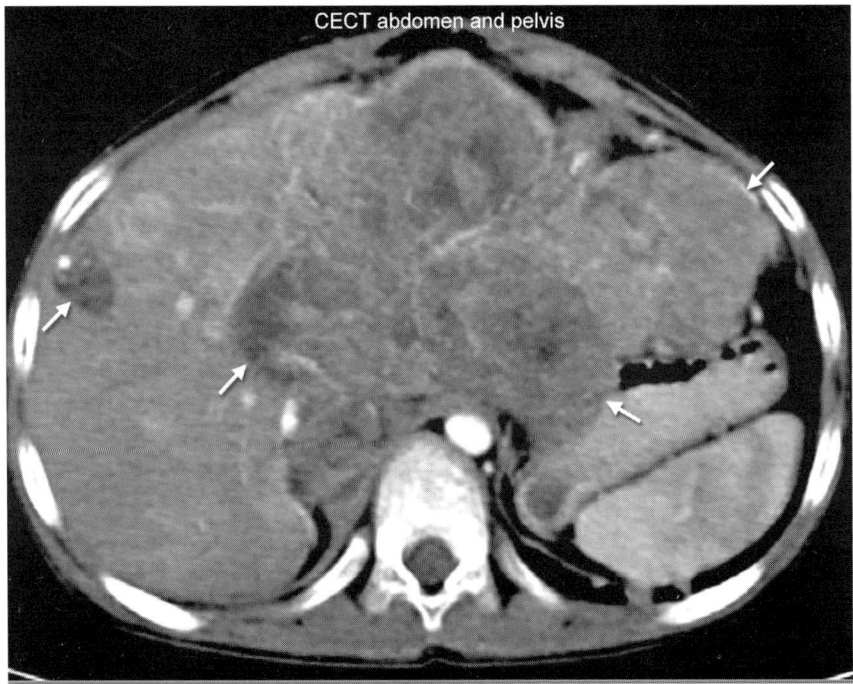

Fig. 1

is hypodense area with calcification in right lobe of liver. This turned out to be hepatoblastoma on histopathological examination.

Comments and Explanation

It is the most common malignant liver tumor in early childhood. On ultrasound, hepatoblastomas appear as predominantly echogenic soft tissue mass. In larger tumors heterogeneity and variable echogenicity is common. Even when large, they tend to be relatively well defined. Intra-lesional calcifications may be visible as areas of shadowing. On CT usually hepatoblastoma appears as a well defined heterogeneous mass, which is usually hypoattenuating compared to surrounding liver. Frequently there are areas of necrosis and hemorrhage. Chunky, dense calcifications may also be seen. CT is also able to evaluate the lungs for metastases and for nodal enlargement. MRI is superior to CT in defining tumor margins, vessel involvement and adenopathy. On T1WI it is generally hypo intense. On GAD, it shows heterogeneous enhancement. On T2WI it is generally hyper intense compared to liver with areas of necrosis and hemorrhages are common.

Opinion

Hepatoblastoma.

Clinical Discussion

Hepatoblastoma primarily affects children from infancy to about 5 years of age. It occurs more frequently in children who were born very prematurely (early) with very low birth weights. Hepatoblastoma is a rare tumor that originates in cells in the liver. Most hepatoblastoma tumors begin in the right lobe of the liver. Hepatoblastoma cancer cells also can spread to other areas of the body. The most common site of metastasis is the lungs. Although the exact cause of liver cancer is unknown, there are a number of genetic conditions that are associated with an increased risk for developing hepatoblastoma. They include: (1) Beckwith-Wiedemann syndrome: this syndrome is characterized by a combination of Wilms' tumor, kidney failure, genitourinary malformations and gonadal (ovaries or testes) abnormalities; (2) Familial adenomatous polyposis and; (3) Gardner syndrome: this is a group of rare inherited diseases of the gastrointestinal tract; (4) Fetal alcohol syndrome; (5) Prematurity and low fetal birth weight; (6) Glycogen storage disease. Children who are exposed to hepatitis B infection at an early age, or those who have biliary atresia, are also at increased risk for developing liver cancer. The signs and symptoms of hepatoblastoma often depend on the size of the tumor and whether it has spread to other parts of the body. Symptoms may include a large mass in the abdomen, weight loss, decreased appetite, vomiting, jaundice, itchy skin and anemia.

CASE 37

Intrahepatic Cholangiocarcinoma

CASE

A 55-year-old male patient came with history of jaundice and pruritus since 15 days and was referred to radiology department for CT scan.

Radiological Findings on CT Examination

Venous phase CT (Fig. 1A) shows patent left portal vein and dilated intrahepatic biliary radicals. No mass is seen. Delayed phase CT (Fig. 1B) shows a vague minimally enhancing mass that was subsequently proven to be a cholangiocarcinoma. Contrast CT (Fig. 1C) in another patient shows dilated intrahepatic biliary radicals in left lobe. No obvious mass is seen. Delayed CT (Fig. 1D) in same patient shows subtle enhancement in mass and thrombosed portal vein.

Comments and Explanation

Cholangiocarcinoma is a malignancy which originates from the intra or extra-hepatic bile duct epithelium. Cholangiocarcinoma is divided into 3 geographic regions—Intrahepatic (least common), Extrahepatic Perihilar (most common, called the Klatskin tumor) and Distal Extrahepatic (Located from the upper border of the pancreas to the ampulla). 95% are Ductal adenocarcinoma, the remainder are squamous cell carcinoma. Intrahepatic cholangiocarcinoma is a carcinoma arising from any portion of the intrahepatic bile duct epithelium. It is the second most common primary intrahepatic malignancy after hepatocellular carcinoma. Many patients present with unresectable or metastatic disease. Preliminary evaluation with positron emission tomography (PET) has shown promise in diagnosing underlying PSC. Small lesions (i.e. <1 cm) have been demonstrated. PET is accurate for detecting nodular carcinomas, but the sensitivity diminishes for infiltrating lesions. PET should be interpreted with caution in patients with PSC and stents in place. PET/CT has been shown to be valuable in detecting unsuspected distant metastasis.

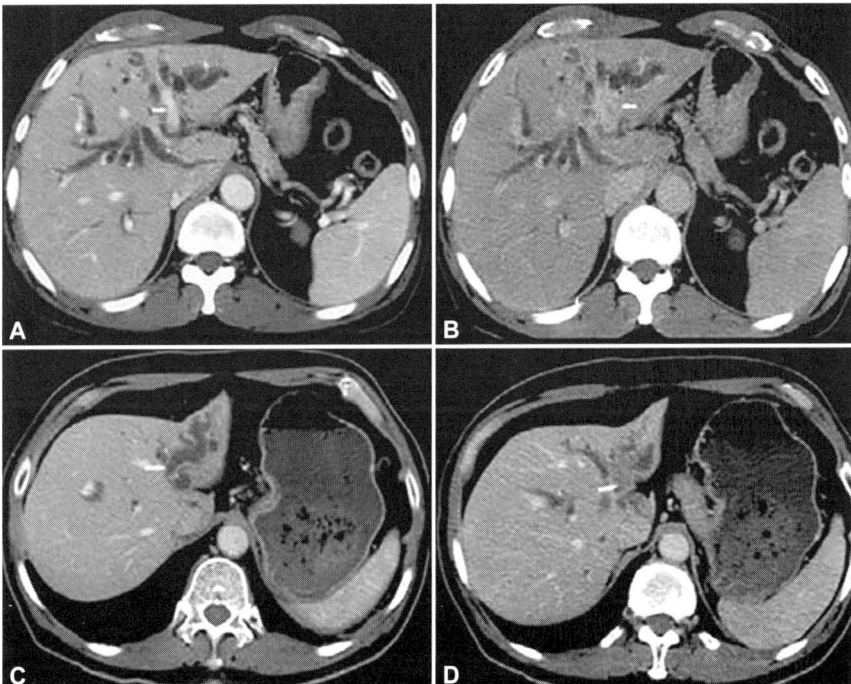

Figs 1A to D

Opinion

Intra-hepatic cholangiocarcinoma.

Clinical Discussion

Cholangiocarcinoma is a biliary duct malignancy that may arise in the liver or in an extrahepatic biliary location. The common manifestation are jaundice, pruritus, weight loss and abdominal pain. The prevalence is higher in men than women. The sixth decade of life is the most common time of presentation. Certain entities have been associated with cholangiocarcinomas. These include infections (liver flukes), chemicals (thorotrast), ulcerative colitis, primary sclerosing cholangitis and Caroli disease. Initially, an ultrasound or CT may be ordered in symptomatic patients. On ultrasound (USG), biliary duct dilatation is the most common finding. The ability to delineate a mass is very variable on USG. Intrahepatic cholangiocarcinomas can be difficult to depict on CT. If seen, the mass is round or oval with segmental biliary dilatation. Delayed contrast enhancement is a typical feature which can help in differentiation from hepatocellular carcinoma. MRI has become the imaging modality of choice. It allows superior evaluation of the liver parenchyma. The mass appears hypointense on T1 weighted images. On T2 images, most masses are isointense or mildly hyperintense. Concentric enhancement is present. Delayed enhancement is a typical feature. Using MRCP, the biliary ducts can be evaluated. MR angiography is useful for staging purposes to exclude vascular involvement. ERCP helps demonstrate the site of biliary obstruction (benign and malignant appearing strictures) using retrograde injection of contrast into the biliary system. Brushings and biopsies can be obtained during the procedure. Stenting as a palliative measure can be offered to help relieve the degree of obstruction. Cholangiocarcinomas tend to grow slowly and to infiltrate the walls of the ducts, dissecting along tissue planes. Local extension occurs into the liver, porta hepatis, and regional lymph nodes of the celiac and pancreaticoduodenal chains. Life-threatening infection (cholangitis) may occur that requires immediate antibiotic intervention and aggressive biliary drainage.

CASE 38

Extrahepatic Cholangiocarcinoma

CASE

Patient came with complain of pain in abdomen, clay colored stool, dark urine since 1 month. Patient was subjected to CT scan abdomen.

Radiological Findings on CT Scan

The intra- and extrahepatic biliary tract and the gallbladder are distended. An enhancing solid mass is seen in the distal end of common bile duct. The biopsy confirmed it as cholangiocarcinoma (Figs 1A to C).

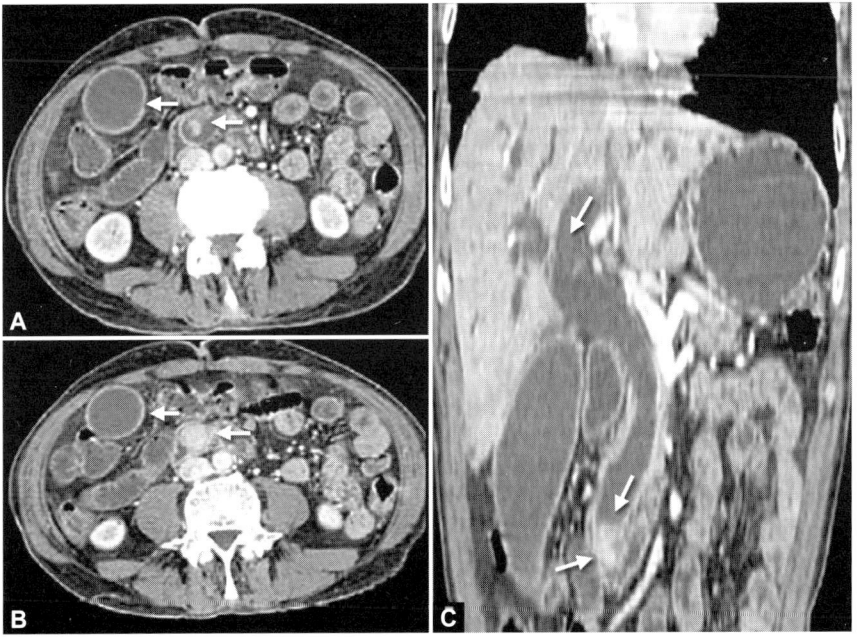

Figs 1A to C

Comments and Explanation

Cholangiocarcinoma is neoplasm originating from intra and extrahepatic bile duct epithelium. Cholangiocarcinomas are classified according to their anatomic location as intrahepatic and extrahepatic. The extrahepatic type including cancers involving the confluence of the right and left hepatic ducts accounts for 80–90% and the intrahepatic type for 5–10% of all cholangiocarcinoma.

Opinion

Extrahepatic cholangiocarcinoma.

Clinical Discussion

Cholangiocarcinomas are malignancies of the biliary duct system that may originate in the liver and extrahepatic bile ducts, which terminate at the ampulla of Vater. Most cholangiocarcinomas remain clinically silent until the advanced stages. Once patients become symptomatic, the clinical presentation is dominated by location of tumor. Symptoms of cholangiocarcinoma include jaundice, clay-colored stools, bilirubinuria (dark urine), pruritus, weight loss, and abdominal pain. Jaundice is the most common manifestation of bile duct cancer and, in general, is best detected in direct sunlight. The obstruction and subsequent cholestasis tend to occur early if the tumor is located in the common bile duct or common hepatic duct. Pruritus usually is preceded by jaundice. Weight loss is a variable finding and may be present in one third of patients at the time of diagnosis. Abdominal pain is relatively common in advanced disease and often is described as a dull ache in the right upper quadrant. Complications include infection, liver failure and spread of tumor to other organs. To afford a chance at cure, complete surgical excision is needed. However, only 10% of patients present early enough to be afforded curative resection. Nonsurgical therapies include stenting and drainage to help improve obstructive symptoms. Chemoradiation therapy is used successfully as adjuvant therapy and to help reduce tumor size prior to surgery. The poorest survival rates are for those individuals with nonresectable disease with palliative stent placement.

CASE 39

Transient Hepatic Attenuation Difference

CASE

A 45-year-old male patient was referred to radiology department for CT scan abdomen.

Radiological Findings on CT Examination

Figures 1A to D transient hepatic attenuation difference (THAD) is an attenuation difference of the liver appearing during bolus-enhanced dynamic CT usually not corresponding to any mass. It is generally seen as an area of high attenuation on the hepatic arterial phase image (A and B) that returns to normal attenuation on the portal venous phase (C and D) images.

Comments and Explanation

The liver has a dual blood supply (70% portal vein, 30% hepatic artery) with compensatory relationships: arterial flow increases when portal flow decreases. Transient hepatic attenuation difference (THAD) is an attenuation difference of the liver appearing during contrast enhanced dynamic CT and not corresponding to mass.

Opinion

Transient hepatic attenuation difference.

Clinical Discussion

Transient hepatic attenuation difference (THAD) is generally seen as an area of high attenuation on the hepatic arterial phase that returns to normal attenuation on the portal venous phase images. According to morphology, they can be divided into four groups (a) Lobar multisegmental; (b) Sectorial; (c) Polymorphous; (d) Diffuse. (a) *Lobar:* They involve almost all segments of one hepatic lobe and are usually caused by an increase in arterial inflow

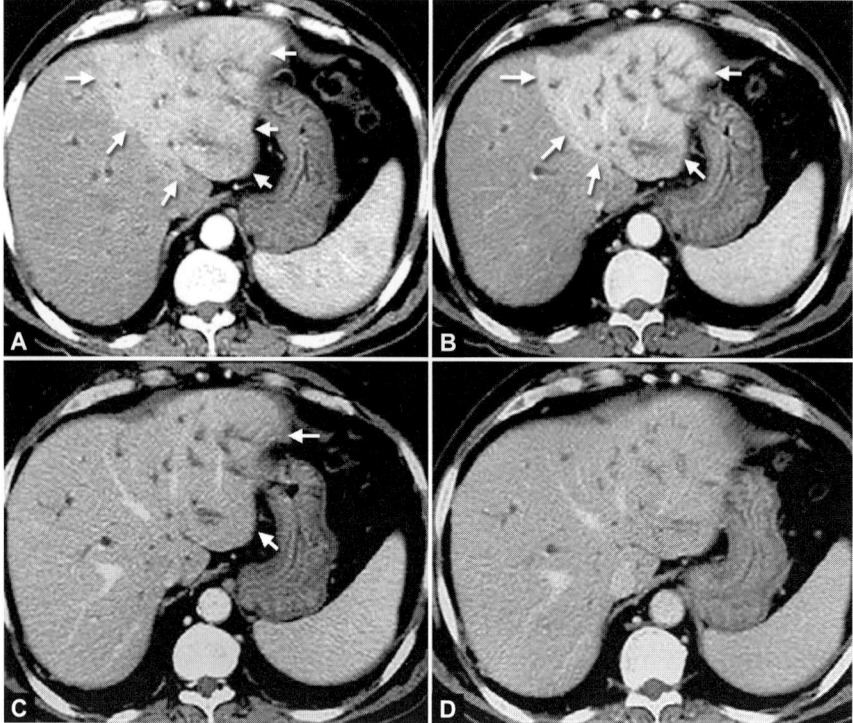

Figs 1A to D

and therefore follow arterial distribution. They usually occur when a hypervascular focal lesion like hepatocellular carcinoma, hemangioma, focal nodular hyperplasia or hypervascular metastases leads to hyperperfusion of the surrounding parenchyma ("siphoning effect") in the absence of portal hypoperfusion. They do not show a triangular shape or a straight border sign; (b) *Sectorial:* They follow portal vein branches, are either wedge or fan-shaped with at least one straight border sign (a clear separation line from the normally attenuating parenchyma) when not associated with focal lesions. They can be caused by portal or hepatic vein thrombosis, long-standing biliary obstruction, or an arterioportal shunt. In such cases, THADs are always wedge-shaped with a straight border sign; (c) *Polymorphous:* Usually does not follow the portal vein branches and show various shapes and sizes without a straight border sign; (d) *Diffuse:* Differences involve the entire hepatic parenchyma and may assume a patchy, central peripheral or peribiliary pattern on the basis of location of the portal blockade. Right heart failure and Budd-Chiari syndrome results in a generalized central lobular enhancement during the arterial phase. When obstruction takes place at the level of portal trunk, as in portal vein thrombosis portal flow remains adequate for central zones of liver but not for the peripheral ones. The arterial response produces enhancement of the peripheral subcapsular hepatic parenchyma with relative hypodensity of the central perihilar area. This CT pattern is called a "central-peripheral" phenomenon.

SECTION 10

Gallbladder

40. Choledochal Cyst
41. Acalculus Cholecystitis
42. Acute Calculus Cholecystitis
43. Emphysematous Cholecystitis
44. Choledocholithiasis
45. Porcelain Gallbladder
46. Carcinoma Gallbladder

CASE 40

Choledochal Cyst

CASE

A 1-year-old female patient with history of jaundice was referred to radiology department for CT scan abdomen.

Radiological Findings on CT Examination

Figures 1A to E: (A) US shows the dilated, tortuous and ectatic left hepatic duct; (B) CECT demonstrates a large cyst lying medial to gallbladder; (C) CECT shows the dilated, tortuous and ectatic left hepatic duct (similar to USG Figure A) with minimal dilatation of intrahepatic biliary radicles; (D) MRI cholangiography shows the cyst medial to the gallbladder with dilated left hepatic duct; (E) Photograph of resected specimen shows choledochal cyst, gallbladder and the cystic duct.

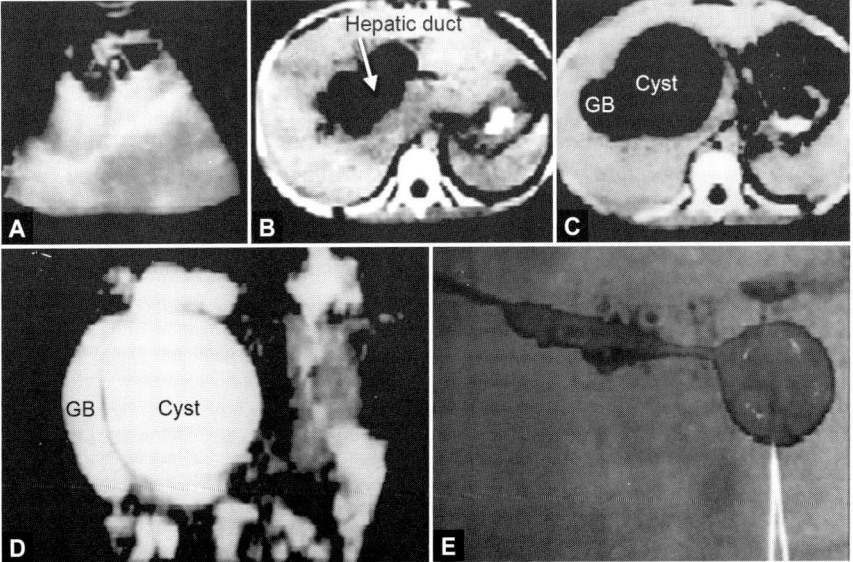

Figs 1A to E *(For color version E, see plate 3)*

Comments and Explanation

Choledochal cysts are unusual congenital anomalies of the biliary tree characterized by cystic dilation of the bile ducts. An anomalous junction of the common bile duct and pancreatic duct proximal to the sphincter of Oddi (outside of the duodenal wall) results in a long common channel of the common bile duct and the pancreatic duct. Because of the long common channel, pancreatic enzymes reflux into the common bile duct when the sphincter of Oddi is contracted. This leads to injury of the biliary wall and results in dilation. This is the major etiologic factor in the development of choledochal cysts.

Opinion

Choledochal cyst.

Clinical Discussion

Choledochal cysts are three times more common in females than males and usually present in childhood. Children or adults with choledochal cysts often present with abdominal pain, jaundice, or a palpable mass The Todani classification system arranges them into 5 basic categories. **Type I** choledochal cyst is a focal, saccular or fusiform dilation of the common bile duct, not extending into the intrahepatic biliary ducts. **Type II** choledochal cyst is a true diverticulum of the common bile duct. **Type III** choledochal cyst is also called a choledochocele. It is a dilation of the most distal intraduodenal portion of the common bile duct. **Type IV** choledochal cysts have multiple intra and extrahepatic biliary duct cysts. **Type V** choledochal cysts refers to Caroli's disease in which there is saccular dilation of the intrahepatic biliary ducts with sparing of the extrahepatic ducts. In infancy, choledochal cysts can lead to biliary obstruction. USG shows a cystic extrahepatic mass. CT shows a dilated cystic mass with distinct walls that is separate from the gallbladder and may appear thickened if there is history of chronic cholangitis. MRI/MRCP shows a large fusiform or extrahepatic mass with strong signal on fluid sensitive sequences and can usually identify the anatomy of the ductal structures. NM hepatobiliary scan shows photopenic defect during initial images with later filling and stasis of radiotracer within cysts. Cholelithiasis, choledocholithiasis, cystolithiasis, cholangitis, biliary cirrhosis, portal hypertension and malignancy are all complications of choledochal cysts. The risk of malignancy increases with age. Treatment is surgical excision with Roux-en-Y hepaticojejunostomy.

CASE 41

Acalculus Cholecystitis

CASE

A middle age male presented to the department of radiology with pain in upper right quadrant of abdomen with nausea and vomiting since last 3 days.

Radiological Findings on CT Examination

CT abdomen (Figs 1A and B) shows thickened edematous gallbladder wall which reveals nodular enhancement. There is stranding of adjacent fat. No evidence of calculus noted. This is suggestive of acalculus cholecystitis.

Comments and Explanation

Acalculus cholecystitis is an acute necroinflammatory disease of the gallbladder with absence of gallbladder calculi. The usual finding on imaging studies is a distended acalculous gallbladder with thickened walls more than 3-4 mm with or without pericholecystic fluid. The diagnosis of acute acalculous cholecystitis with CT requires that 2 major diagnostic criteria be met or, alternatively, that 1 major criterion and 2 minor criteria be met. These criteria are as follows:

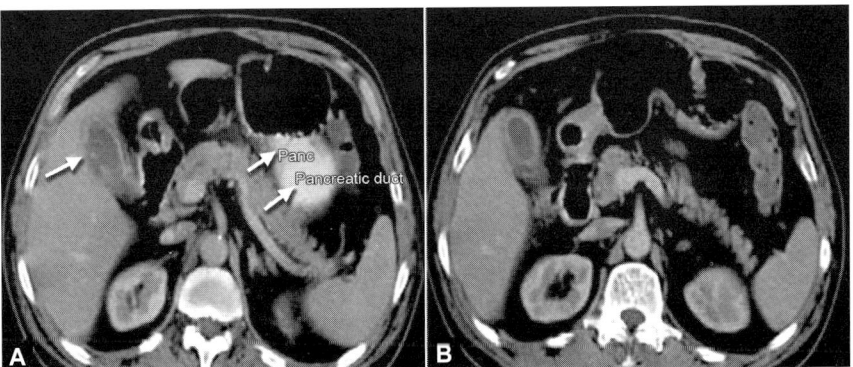

Figs 1A and B

Major Criteria

- Gallbladder wall thickening greater than 3 mm
- Subserosal halo (i.e. gallbladder wall edema)
- Pericholecystic fatty inflammation
- Pericholecystic fluid (without ascites or hypoalbuminemia)
- Mucosal sloughing
- Intramural gas.

Minor Criteria

- Gallbladder distention (>5 cm transverse)
- High-attenuation bile (sludge).

Opinion

Acute acalculus cholecystitis.

Clinical Discussion

Acalculous cholecystitis is typically seen in patients who are hospitalized and critically ill, though it may also be seen in the outpatient setting. It is a potentially fatal form of acute cholecystitis that usually occurs in critically ill patients. The disease may often go unrecognized due to the complexity of the patient's medical and surgical problems. It has also been found in association with total parenteral nutrition, mechanical ventilation, and the use of narcotic analgesics, as well as in major cardiovascular disorders, complicated diabetes mellitus, autoimmune disease, AIDS and bile stasis. Complications include perforation or rupture. Ischemia/reperfusion injury to the gallbladder is a central pathogenic feature.

CASE 42

Acute Calculus Cholecystitis

CASE

A middle age man presented with complaints of abdominal pain for 4 days which was localized to epigastric region with radiation to right upper quadrant.

Radiological Finding on CT Examination

CT scan shows multiple hyperdense calculi of varying sizes in gallbladder lumen. There is pericholecystic collection (Fig. 1).

In another case CT images show distended gallbladder (GB) with multiple hyperdense calculi and thickened wall especially in the region of fundus

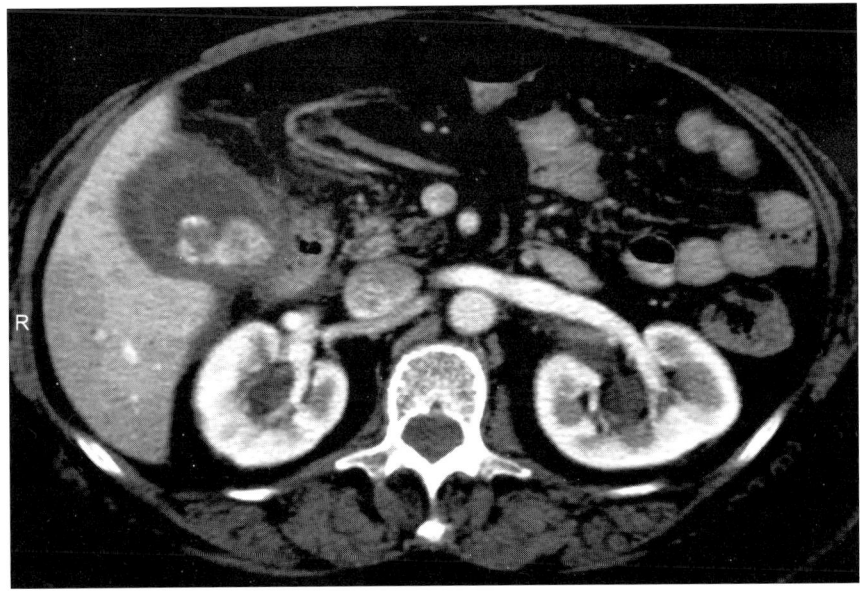

Fig. 1

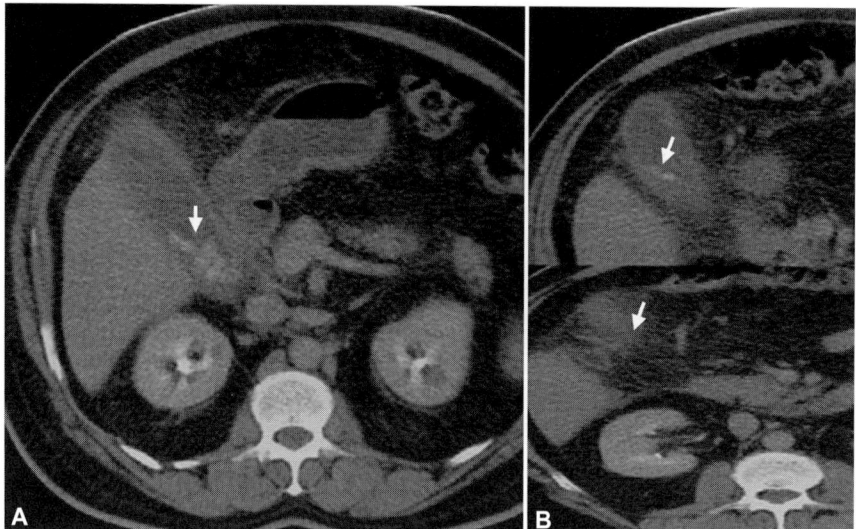

Figs 2A and B

associated with soft tissue stranding in the adjacent greater omental fat in a case of cholelithiasis with acute cholecystitis (Figs 2A and B).

Comments and Explanation

Cholecystitis is inflammation of gallbladder. It may be associated with gallstones or, less often, without gallstones (acalculous cholecystitis). It can be acute or chronic. Acute calculus cholecystitis results from gallbladder stones. It occurs when a stone blocks the cystic duct, which carries bile from the gallbladder. Plain X-ray abdomen may show radio-opacities in right hypochondriac region. Ultrasound shows an obstructing gallstone, dilatation of the GB, a positive sonographic Murphy's sign (i.e. pain elicited by pressure over the sonographically located gallbladder), pericholecystic fat inflammation or fluid and hyperemia of the GB wall at power Doppler.

CT scan findings include gallstones within the GB, the cystic duct, or both; more than 3 mm of focal or diffuse thickening of the GB wall in a noncontracted GB; indistinct liver-GB interface; fluid in the GB fossa in the absence of ascites; enlargement of the GB, with the transverse diameter measuring more than 5 cm; infiltration of the surrounding fat; increased bile attenuation, caused by biliary sludge.

Opinion

Acute calculus cholecystitis.

Clinical Discussion

Acute calculus cholecystitis is a common disease. A typical presentation is several hours of progressively worsening right upper quadrant pain, followed by nausea and vomiting. Often, the patient has had repeated similar episodes in the past. These symptoms are caused by gallstone lodging in the neck of the GB or the cystic duct, resulting in biliary stasis. Although the cause is not believed to be primarily infectious, after the stone has caused biliary obstruction, superinfection is a common occurrence without treatment. If the diagnosis is suspected clinically, ultrasound is the imaging modality of choice.

CASE 43

Emphysematous Cholecystitis

CASE

A 63-year-old diabetic male presented to the department of radiology with history of right hypochondriac pain.

Radiological Findings on CT Examination

Contrast enhanced axial CT images at the level of pancreas show presence of air in the gallbladder wall and lumen, common bile duct and pancreatic duct (Fig. 1).

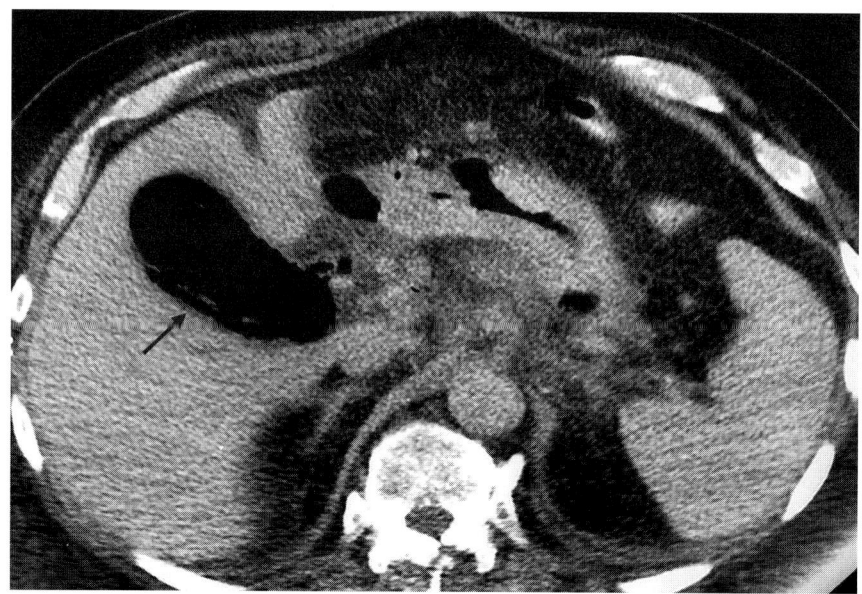

Fig. 1

Comments and Explanation

Emphysematous cholecystitis is an acute infection of the gallbladder wall caused by gas-forming organisms that is considered a surgical emergency. Usually, the diagnosis is made by the radiographic presence of air within the wall or lumen of gallbladder. On USG intramural gas appears as an arclike echogenic interface with posterior reverberation artefact. CT demonstrates emphysematous changes in the gallbladder wall that are diagnostic of this condition and is highly sensitive for tiny bubbles of air which may not be seen on ultrasonography. CT is considered the most sensitive and specific imaging modality for identifying gas within the gallbladder lumen or wall. The presence of pneumoperitoneum indicates perforation. CT scanning can also provide precise information regarding the location and extent of air and fluid collections, such as extension into the pericholecystic tissues and the hepatic ducts. The radiologic differential diagnosis is that presence of gas in the biliary tree, which may be due to a biliary-enteric fistula, following ERCP; or may be due to cholangitis caused by gas-forming organisms.

Opinion

Emphysematous cholecystitis.

Clinical Discussion

Emphysematous cholecystitis is an uncommon, insidious, and rapidly progressive form of acute cholecystitis, characterized by early gangrene, perforation of the gallbladder and high mortality. Most of the patients are males between 50 and 70 years of age and have underlying diabetes mellitus and peripheral atherosclerotic disease. The most common clinical complaints initially are right upper quadrant pain and fever. The insidious nature of this disease may mislead the clinician, and the patient may unsuspectingly rapidly deteriorate with sudden cardiovascular collapse and even death. Prompt surgical cholecystectomy, with excision of the gallbladder is the mainstay of treatment because of the observation that septic shock and death progresses quickly with this disease process, particularly in the elderly and diabetic individuals.

CASE 44

Choledocholithiasis

CASE

A 48-year-old male patient presented to the department of radiology with history of pain in right side of upper abdomen since one month with yellowish discolouration of skin since 10 days for CT abdomen.

Radiological Findings on CT Examination

Plain CT images show massive dilatation of intrahepatic biliary radicals and common bile duct (Figs 1A and B) secondary to an intraluminal calculus in distal common bile duct (Figs 1C and D).

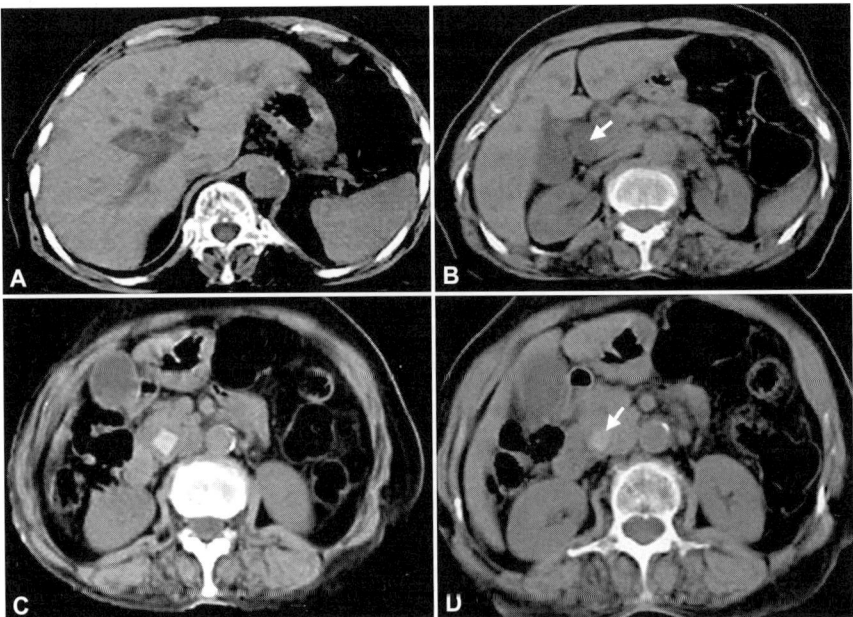

Figs 1A to D

Comment and Explanation

Cholesterol or black pigment stones are more likely to form in the gallbladder, while almost all brown pigment stones form in the bile duct. A classic ultrasound finding with calcified stones is posterior acoustic shadowing, however, the appearance of gallstones is based upon the location, size, and composition. The best imaging tools to evaluate choledocholithiasis is ultrasound or magnetic resonance cholangiopancreatography (MRCP). Conventional CT is useful for detecting central round dense stone, target sign, surrounding hypodense mucosa, calcified stone, hypodense bile surrounding calculus like a crescent, biliary dilatation. MRCP shows filling defects within biliary tree on T2W images. There are narrow differential for CBD calculus and depend on modality. Differentials include cholangiocarcinoma, carcinoma of ampulla of Vater, pancreatic carcinoma; parasites. Artefacts like air bubbles, susceptibility artefacts, flow voids, vascular impression, and sphincter contractions can be mistaken as CBD calculi.

Opinion

Choledocholithiasis.

Clinical Discussion

Stones within the bile duct may form either *in situ* or pass from the gallbladder, and when recurrent tend to be pigment stones. Stone in bile duct does not cause discomfort to patient but when blockage becomes severe patient may experience abdominal pain in right upper abdomen, fever, nausea, vomiting and loss of appetite. When a gallstone is stuck in the bile duct, the bile can become infected. The presence of parasitic infection of *Ascaris lumbricoides* or *Clonorchis sinensis* may result in formation of CBD stone due to ductal inflammation, proximal stasis. It can move into the ductal system and then into the liver. It can become a life-threatening infection. Possible complications include infection, biliary cirrhosis, cholangitis, pancreatitis, gallbladder carcinoma, gallbladder polyp, primary sclerosing cholangitis, and porcelain gallbladder.

CASE 45

Porcelain Gallbladder

CASE

A 40-year-old male patient with history of intense pain in the upper-right side of the abdomen with nausea and vomiting, was referred to radiology department for CT abdomen.

Radiological Findings on CT Examination

Plain CT abdomen (Fig. 1A) shows hyperdense appearance in the dependent part of gallbladder due to multiple small calculi. There is calcification of the wall (porcelain gallbladder). In right lateral decubitus position the calculi have shifted to the now dependent position (Fig. 1B).

Comment and Explanation

Cholelithiasis is defined as calculi in gallbladder. Porcelain gallbladder means the wall of the gallbladder has been calcified to hard bluish white texture resembling

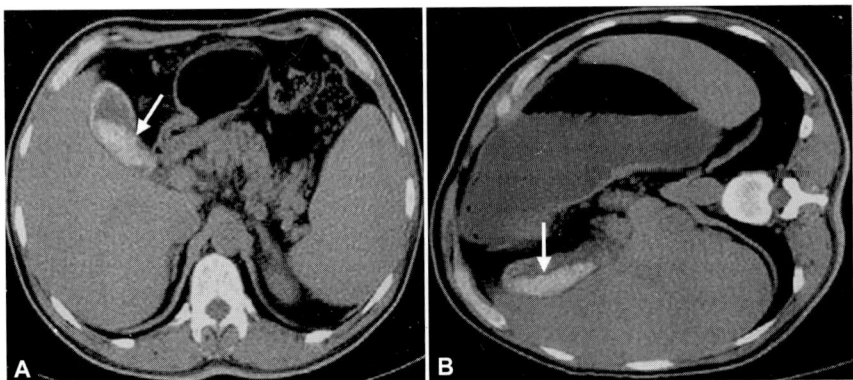

Figs 1A and B

porcelain ceramic. This medical condition primarily results from a chronically inflamed organ (Figs 1A and B).

Opinion

Cholelithiasis in porcelain gallbladder.

Clinical Discussion

Most people with cholelithiasis have no symptoms at all. A minority of patients with gallstones develop symptoms: severe abdominal pain, nausea and vomiting, and complete blockage of the bile ducts that may pose the risk of infection.

Extensive calcium encrustation of the gallbladder wall has been termed calcified gallbladder, calcifying cholecystitis, or cholecystopathia chronica calcarea. The term "porcelain gallbladder" has been used to emphasize the blue discoloration and brittle consistency of the gallbladder wall at surgery. When complete wall of gallbladder is calcified it is called porcelain gallbladder. Calcification in the right upper quadrant of the abdomen has several causes. Porcelain gallbladder must be differentiated from large solitary calcified gallstones, which are seldom as large as porcelain gallbladders.

Calcification of the gallbladder wall or milk-of-calcium bile may have identical appearances on sonograms; therefore, sometimes plain radiography is important in distinguishing these entities.

Emphysematous cholecystitis can mimic porcelain gallbladder on sonograms; however, their clinical presentation is distinct from that of porcelain gallbladder. Complications include cholecystitis, Mirizzi syndrome, and cholecystocholedochal fistula and gallstone ileus.

CASE 46

Carcinoma Gallbladder

CASE

A 70-year-old male with history of pain in abdomen, nausea and vomiting was referred to the department of radiology for CT abdomen and pelvis.

Radiological Findings on CT Examination

Contrast enhanced CT abdomen (Fig. 1) shows a lobulated soft tissue density enhancing lesion seen in lumen extending to the neck of the gallbladder (white arrow). Enlarged necrotic lymph nodes are seen in precaval and retrocaval regions (black arrows).

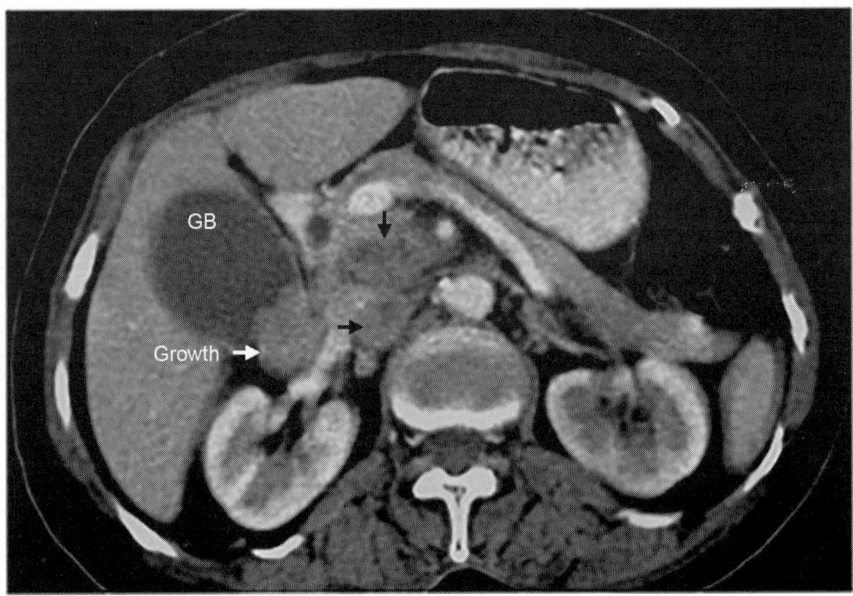

Fig. 1

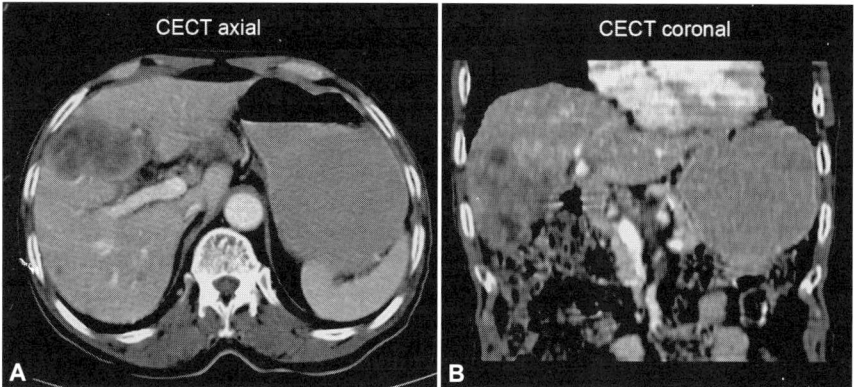

Figs 2A and B

In another case CECT abdomen (Figs 2A and B) show a large heterogeneously enhancing lesion replacing the entire gallbladder and infiltrating into the adjacent liver parenchyma.

Comments and Explanation

Carcinoma of gallbladder is the most common malignant tumor of biliary tract. Ultrasound shows heterogeneous mass in sub hepatic space replacing the GB. Gallbladder carcinoma may be seen as an intraluminal fungating mass with diffuse thickening of wall with or without cholelithiasis. The tumor mass may contain low-attenuation areas of necrosis. Use of contrast-enhanced CT is extremely helpful for distinguishing complicated cholecystitis from gallbladder carcinoma. The CT demonstration of associated lymphadenopathy, soft-tissue extension into the liver, and evidence of hematogenous metastases favors the diagnosis of gallbladder carcinoma. Additional CT findings can include extrahepatic biliary duct obstruction due to metastasis to pericholedochal and superior pancreaticoduodenal nodes, encasement of common bile duct, biliary dilatation and involvement of adjacent structures like liver. The most common mode by which gallbladder carcinoma spreads to adjacent organs is direct extension, followed by lymphatic and vascular extension. Intraperitoneal and intraductal spread of tumor also occur. The liver is the organ most frequently involved by direct contiguous spread, followed by the colon, duodenum and pancreas. Without other primary or secondary tumors, local recurrence or distant metastases are visualized with positron emission tomography on the basis of increased fluorodeoxyglucose uptake.

Opinion

Gallbladder carcinoma.

Clinical Discussion

The clinical features of gallbladder carcinoma include right upper quadrant pain, anorexia, weight loss, and jaundice. Often, the patient's condition is clinically indistinguishable from that seen in acute or chronic cholecystitis. Although the presence of cholelithiasis is not correlated with gallbladder carcinoma, the prevalence of cholelithiasis in cases of gallbladder carcinoma has been previously reported to be in the range of 80-90%. Porcelain gallbladder is complicated by gallbladder carcinoma in up to 25% of cases. Over 90% of cases of gallbladder cancer are adenocarcinoma. Unfortunately, due to the largely asymptomatic nature of these tumors, presentation is typically late with the majority of tumors being large, unresectable, with direct extension into adjacent structures or distant metastases present at diagnosis. Curative resection is only possible for localized early disease, which is usually found incidentally.

SECTION 11

Pancreas

47. Acute Pancreatitis
48. Pancreatic Pseudocyst
49. Necrotizing Pancreatitis
50. Periampullary Carcinoma with Metastases

CASE 47

Acute Pancreatitis

CASE

A 40-year-old male with severe epigastric pain and raised serum lipase levels was referred to the department of radiology for CT scan abdomen.

Radiological Findings on CT Examination

CT abdomen reveals bilateral pleural effusions (Fig. 1A) and bulky edematous pancreas (Fig. 1B). Thin walled encapsulated fluid collections are seen in the region of stomach bed, anterior to pancreas extending inferior to tail of pancreas and anterior to Gerota's fascia (Figs 1B to D).

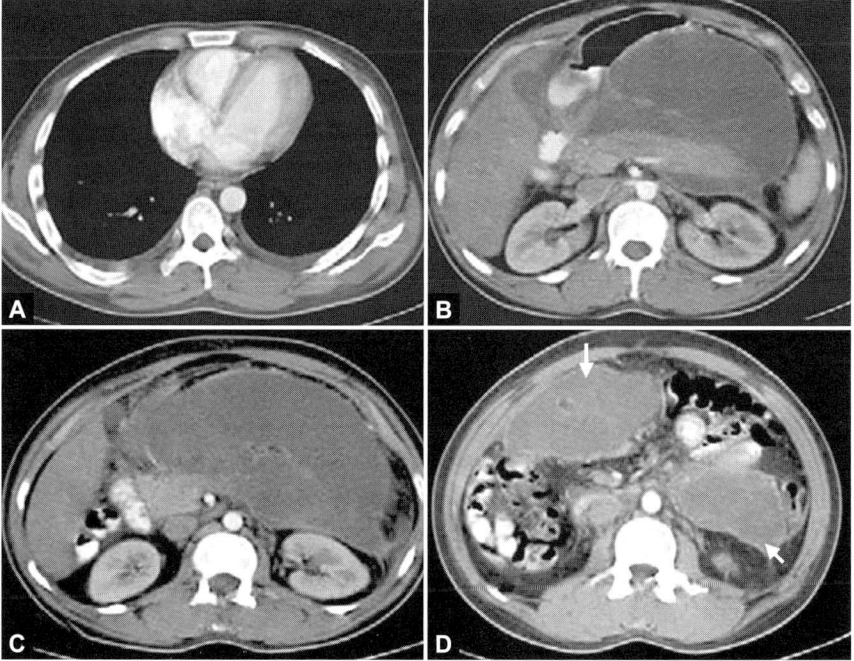

Figs 1A to D

Comments and Explanation

Acute pancreatitis is defined as an acute inflammatory process of the pancreas with variable involvement of other regional tissues or remote organ systems. Contrast enhanced CT is the standard imaging modality for evaluating acute pancreatitis and its complications. Intra-abdominal fluid collections and collections of necrotic tissue are common in acute pancreatitis. In the early stage these collections do not have a wall or capsule. Preferred locations are the omental bursa and the retroperitoneal space (anterior and posterior pararenal space).These collections are the result of the release of activated pancreatic enzymes namely lipase and amylase which cause necrosis of the surrounding tissues. Abnormalities seen in pancreas include focal or diffuse parenchymal enlargement, indistinctness of the margins of the gland due to inflammation and surrounding retroperitoneal fat stranding. Infected necrosis of pancreatic parenchyma and/or extrapancreatic fatty tissue can also be seen. Air bubbles are seen in patients with infected necrosis.

Balthazar score is used in CT severity index (CTSI) for grading of acute pancreatitis. It is as follows:
- *Normal pancreas:* Score 0
- *Enlargement of pancreas:* Score 1
- *Inflammatory changes in pancreas and peripancreatic fat:* Score 2
- *Ill defined single fluid collection:* Score 3
- *Two or more poorly defined fluid collections:* Score 4

The extent of pancreatic necrosis is graded as follows:
- *Score 0:* None
- *Score 2:* Less than/equal to 30%
- *Score 4:* > 30–50%
- *Score 6:* > 50%

Opinion

Acute pancreatitis.

Clinical Discussion

Gallstones and alcohol abuse are the most common causes of acute pancreatitis. Other causes include blunt trauma to the abdomen, drug-induced, infectious etiologies (e.g. mumps, cytomegalovirus) and congenital anomalies like pancreas divisum. Local complications of acute pancreatitis include fluid collections, pseudocyst formation, abscess, pancreatic necrosis and hemorrhage. Pseudocyst is a collection of pancreatic juice enclosed by a wall of fibrous tissue. It requires 4 or more weeks to develop and there is often communication with the pancreatic duct. Pancreatitis and pseudocysts can cause a number of vascular complications such as vascular occlusion, pseudoaneurysm and spontaneous hemorrhage. Pseudoaneurysm can occur in any vessel in the peripancreatic area but the most common vessel is the splenic artery.

CASE 48

Pancreatic Pseudocyst

CASE

A 25-year-old male with history of pancreatitis was referred to radiology department for CT scan abdomen.

Radiological Findings on CT Examination

Contrast enhanced CT scan abdomen shows a well defined cyst in the region of body and tail of pancreas. It has a thin peripherally enhancing wall (Fig. 1A). No septation or solid components seen within it, this represents a pseudocyst. The head of the pancreas appears normal (Fig. 1B).

In Other Cases

- Contrast enhanced CT scan abdomen (Fig. 2A) shows peripherally enhancing loculated collection in the retrocardiac region. Bilateral pleural effusion is seen. Another well defined cystic lesion with a thin peripherally enhancing wall is seen in left posterior pararenal space pushing the left kidney antero-laterally. This represents a pseudocyst (Fig. 2B). Also a loculated mesenteric collection is seen in left side of abdomen (Fig. 2C).

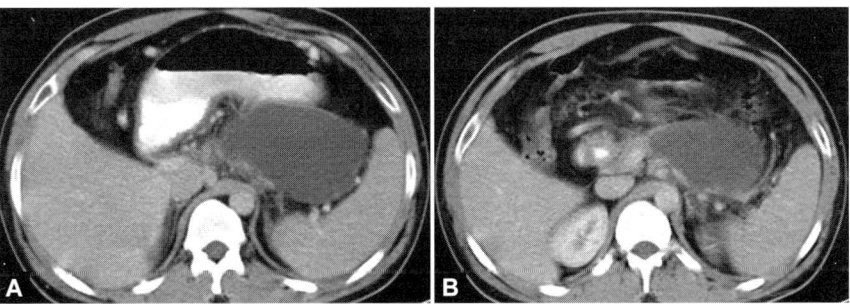

Figs 1A and B

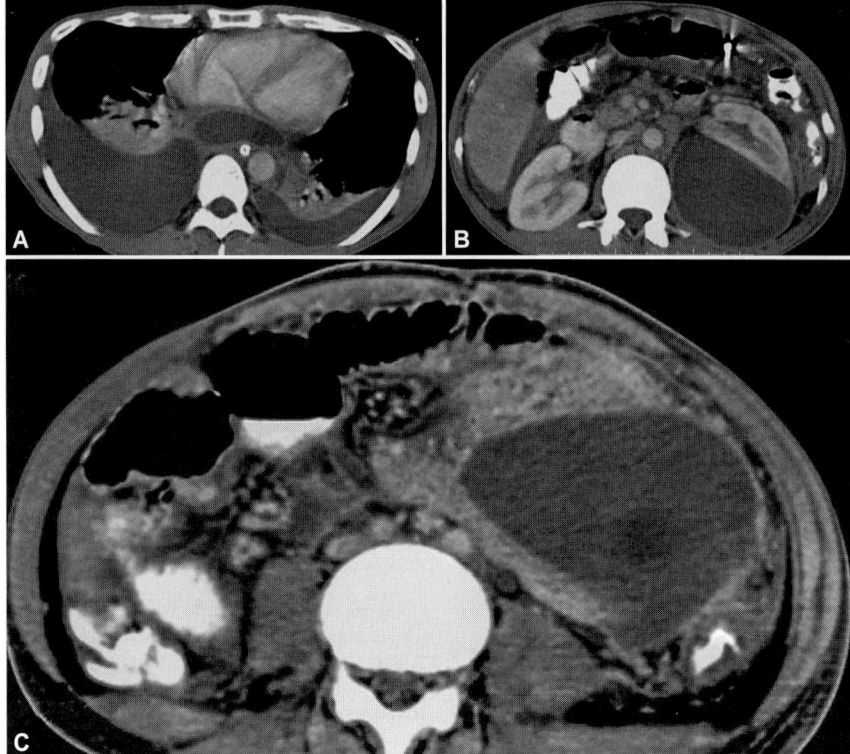

Figs 2A to C

- Axial post contrast CT image of abdomen at the level of pancreas (Fig. 3) shows a well defined cystic lesion arising from the anterior portion of body of pancreas with irregular margin. There is evidence of air fluid level within it. This represents an infected pseudocyst of pancreas. Also there is peripancreatic fat stranding and the head of pancreas appears bulky.

Comments and Explanation

Excessive alcohol consumption is most common cause of pancreatitis. Abdominal CT scanning is an excellent choice for imaging of pancreatic pseudocysts. Presentations attributed to pseudocyst include mass effect leading to biliary obstruction or gastric outlet obstruction. Pseudocysts are fluid filled oval or round collections with a relatively thick wall. They can be multiple and are most commonly located in the pancreatic bed. However, they can be found anywhere from the groin to the mediastinum and even in the neck, having ascended in the retroperitoneum via the diaphragmatic hiatus into the mediastinum. CT attenuation values may be greater than 20–30 Hounsfield units because of the presence of necrotic pancreatic or peripancreatic debris. The presence of such

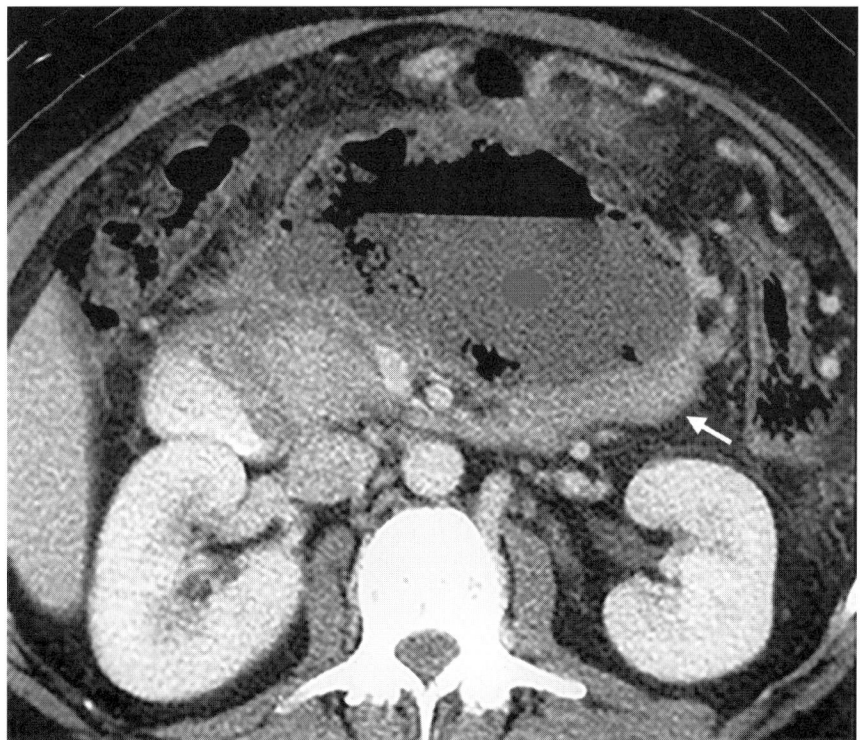

Fig. 3

material in the pseudocyst makes its appearance more heterogeneous on CT scans. Pancreatic pseudocysts have several features that help to distinguish them from acute fluid collections on CT scans. Most prominent is the presence of a well-defined, nonepithelial, fibrous wall around the collection. Pseudocysts are round or ovoid in configuration with an enhancing wall whereas acute fluid collections are not well defined. It develops in 4–6 weeks, usually decreases in size over time, sometimes enlarges or become infected. When it becomes infected there is evidence of air pockets or air fluid level within the cyst. The major weakness of CT scanning is the inability to distinguish pseudocyst from cystic neoplasms, especially mucinous cystadenomas and intraductal papillary mucinous tumors (IPMT). The clinical history provides clue to a diagnosis other than pancreatic pseudocyst. If the patient has had no prior history of pancreatitis but has a cystic mass associated with the pancreas, an alternative diagnosis should be considered.

Opinion

Pancreatic pseudocysts.

Clinical Discussion

Patient clinically presents as acute pain in epigastric region and high grade fever. There is evidence of history of chronic alcoholism. Pancreatitis leads to formation of pseudocysts. Pseudocyst gets infected and leads to formation of air pockets within. Also peripancreatic fat stranding is seen. Infection occurs either spontaneously or after therapeutic or diagnostic manipulations. While infected pseudocyst can initially be treated with conservative means, a majority of patients will require intervention. Traditionally, surgery has been the preferred modality but endoscopic treatment is gaining acceptance. An external drainage may be necessary in selected situations such as when there is evidence of gross sepsis and the patient is too unstable to undergo surgical or endoscopic drainage.

CASE 49

Necrotizing Pancreatitis

CASE

A middle aged male presented to the department of radiology with history of sudden pain in the upper abdomen which is worse when lying down but may feel less intense when sitting up or bending over since 2 days. Patient also had nausea, vomiting and fever since 4 days.

Radiological Findings on CT Examination

Axial post contrast CT image at the level of pancreas (Fig. 1) shows nonenhancing hypodense area involving the body and tail of pancreas suggesting area of

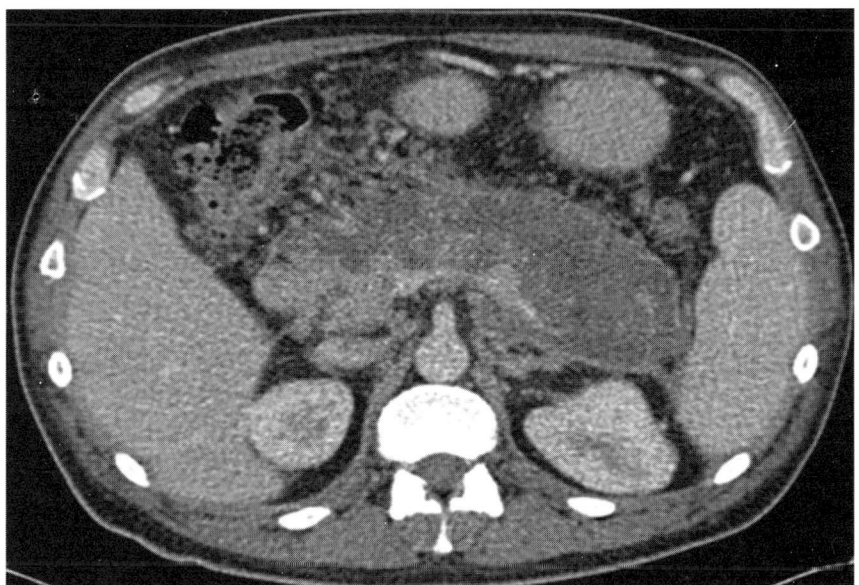

Fig. 1

necrosis along with peripancreatic fat stranding. Findings suggest necrotizing pancreatitis.

Comments and Explanation

Necrotizing pancreatitis represents the severe form of pancreatitis. Pancreatic necrosis is diagnosed radiographically by dynamic intravenous contrast-enhanced computed tomography (CT) of the abdomen. Because the normal pancreatic microcirculation is disrupted during acute necrotizing pancreatitis, affected portions of the pancreas do not show normal contrast enhancement. Contrast-enhanced abdominal CT is the gold standard for the noninvasive diagnosis of pancreatic necrosis, with an accuracy of more than 90%.

Atlanta classification for acute pancreatitis was modified to update the terminology and provide simple functional clinical and morphologic classifications. The modification divides acute pancreatitis into interstitial edematous pancreatitis and necrotizing pancreatitis, distinguish an early phase (1st week) and a late phase (after the 1st week), and emphasize systemic inflammatory response syndrome and multisystem organ failure. In the 1st week, only clinical parameters are important for treatment planning. After the 1st week, morphologic criteria defined on the basis of CT findings combined with clinical parameters form basis for treatment. This revised classification introduces new terminology for pancreatic fluid collections. Depending on presence or absence of necrosis, acute collections in the first 4 weeks are called acute necrotic collections or acute peripancreatic fluid collections. Once an enhancing capsule develops with persistent peripancreatic fluid collections are referred to as pseudocysts; and acute necrotic collections, as walled-off necroses.

Opinion

Necrotizing pancreatitis.

Clinical Discussion

Severe acute pancreatitis is usually a result of pancreatic glandular necrosis. The morbidity and mortality associated with acute pancreatitis are substantially higher when necrosis is present, especially when the area of necrosis is also infected. It is important to identify patients with pancreatic necrosis so that appropriate management can be undertaken. Advances in radiologic imaging and aggressive medical management with emphasis on the prevention of infection have allowed prompt identification of complications and improvement in outcome for necrotizing pancreatitis patients. As long as acute necrotizing pancreatitis remains sterile, the overall mortality is approximately 10%. The mortality rate at least triples if there is infected necrosis. In addition, patients with sterile necrosis and high severity of illness scores accompanied by multisystem organ failure, shock, or renal insufficiency have significantly higher mortality. Complications include pseudocyst of pancreas, pancreatic abscess and sepsis.

CASE 50

Periampullary Carcinoma with Metastases

CASE

A 48-year-old female with history of Whipple's surgery for periampullary carcinoma with referred to the Department of Radiology for a follow-up CT scan.

Radiological Findings on CT Examination

Axial post contrast CT images of abdomen shows an ill defined, hypodense, non-enhancing lesion in segment IV of liver (Fig. 1A) and another similar lesion is seen in segment VII (Fig. 1B). Preaortic and aortocaval lymphadenopathy with central necrosis (Fig. 1C). Figure 1D shows pancreatic duct stent and its drainage into the jejunum (post Whipple's surgery). In an operated case of periampullary carcinoma lesions in liver and enlarged retroperitoneal lymph nodes represent metastases.

Comments and Explanation

Periampullary carcinomas arise within 2 cm of the major papilla in the duodenum and include four different types of malignancies, namely, those originating from (a) the ampulla of Vater itself; (b) the intrapancreatic distal bile duct; (c) the head and uncinate process of the pancreas; and (d) the duodenum.

Accurate diagnosis and origin determination may influence treatment planning and the prediction of prognosis. In comparison to pancreatic cancer, distal bile duct cancer is more resectable. To improve survival, the radical resection of pancreatic cancer should be more frequently combined with chemoradiation therapy or more extensive regional lymphadenectomy than the radical resection of nonpancreatic periampullary cancers. Aggressive resection is indicated in ampullary or duodenal carcinoma, even in the presence of positive lymph nodes at preoperative imaging.

Most complications of pancreatoduodenectomy are managed without radiologic intervention, although many are demonstrated at imaging. These complications include delayed gastric emptying, pancreatic fistula, wound

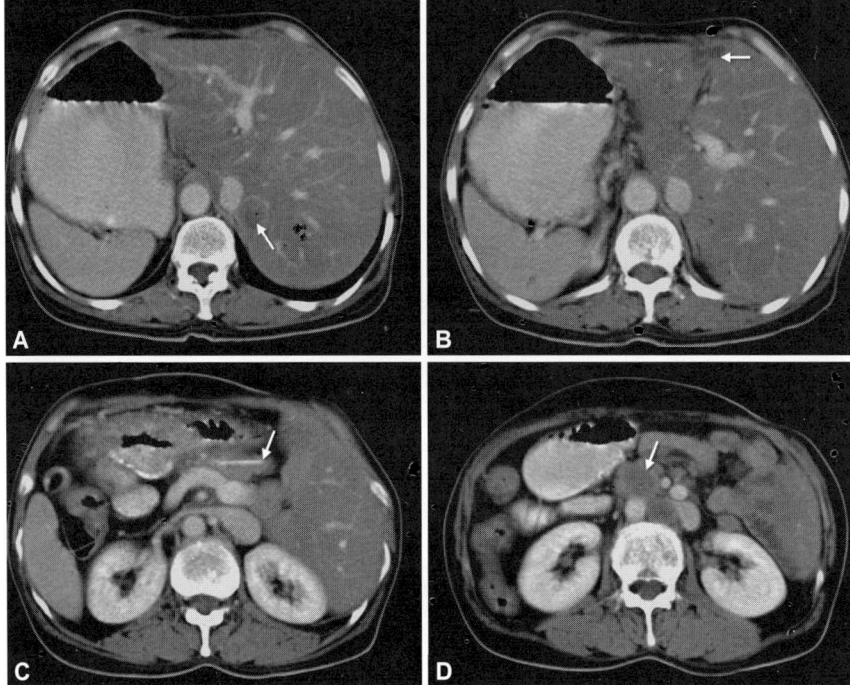

Figs 1A to D

infection, hemorrhage, and pancreatitis. Knowledge of the postoperative anatomy, familiarity with the various CT appearances of a normal loop, and careful evaluation of the loop and its surroundings usually allow definitive diagnosis of the presence or absence of an adjacent abscess. Postoperative abscesses may occur in the retroperitoneal surgical bed or in the peritoneum. The peritoneum allows fluid to migrate easily, and collections can be found remote from the surgical site. One additional interpretive pitfall is a collection in the gallbladder fossa that may mimic the appearance of the gallbladder. This finding should not be misinterpreted as the gallbladder because the gallbladder is usually removed during pancreatoduodenectomy. The bile ducts are very sensitive to ischemia, and violation of the integrity of the intrahepatic bile ducts may result in hepatic abscess or intrahepatic biloma. Biliary obstruction in a patient after pancreatoduodenectomy can result from recurrent tumor, anastomotic stricture, or bile duct injury.

Opinion

Operated case of periampullary carcinoma with hepatic metastases and retroperitoneal lymphadenopathy.

Clinical Discussion

Periampullary tumors, compared to others in the vicinity, are diagnosed and possibly detected early on account of their anatomical location. However, there is a lack of adequate data to support this hypothesis. Thus the main feature is painless progressive jaundice and significant weight loss. Abdominal pain is seen in advanced stages of the disease. Icterus, pruritus, hepatomegaly and a palpable gallbladder are among the prominent clinical features. The combination of MRCP with conventional T1- and T2-weighted MR imaging, including gadolinium-enhanced dynamic MR imaging, is important for the evaluation of periampullary disease in terms of both detection and evaluation of the extent of a periampullary mass.

SECTION 12

Spleen

51. Splenunculus
52. Splenic Trauma
53. Splenic Abscess

CASE 51

Splenunculus

CASE

A 26-year-old male came for routine CT abdomen.

Radiological Findings on CT Scan Examination

Plain and contrast enhanced CT images (Figs 1A and B) show a well defined oval structure medial to the spleen. It shows density and enhancement similar to the spleen on plain and post contrast images. This represents splenunculus.

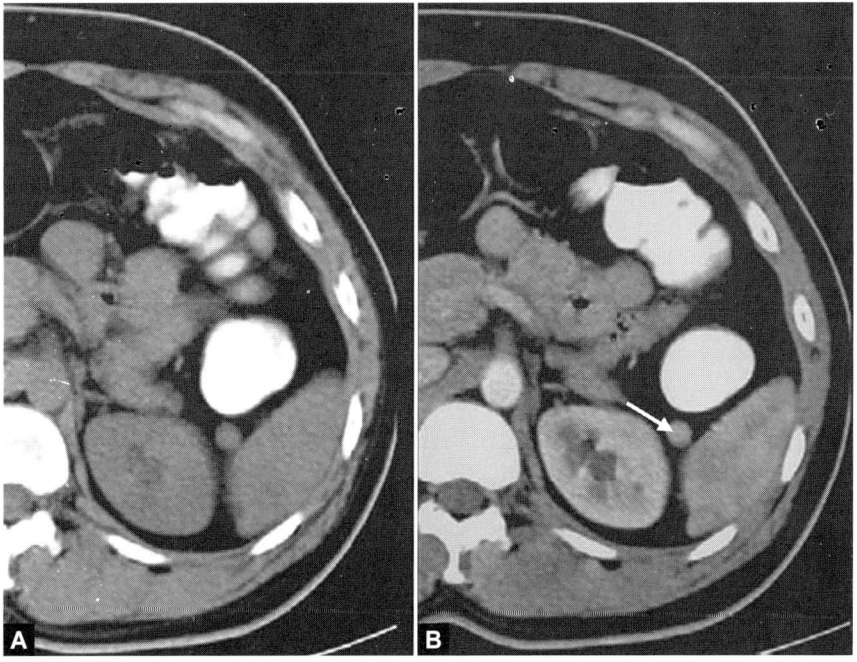

Figs 1A and B

Comments and Explanation

Splenunculus is accessory spleen, generally lies along the splenic artery, near the hilum, or in the omental ligaments around the spleen. Splenunculi occur in normal people and sometimes enlarge following splenectomy.

Opinion

Splenunculus.

Clinical Discussion

Splenunculi are small nodules of spleen that are detached from the rest of the organ. They are benign and asymptomatic, their importance mainly related to the need to distinguish them from more sinister pathology. Splenunculi are typically a few centimeters in diameter when identified, well circumscribed rounded or ovoid nodules. Although most are located near the spleen, they have been identified elsewhere in the abdominal cavity including—near the spleen (the most common), gastrosplenic ligament, splenorenal ligament, pancreatic tail, greater omentum, mesentery, stomach or bowel wall. They have density and enhancing characteristics similar to the rest of the spleen on CT. General imaging differential considerations include peritoneal metastases, enlarged lymph node and tumor from the tail of pancreas.

CASE 52

Splenic Trauma

CASE

A 62-year-old male patient came with history of road traffic accident and pain in left side of abdomen. CT was done to rule out abdominal organ injury.

Radiological Findings on CT Examination

There is crescentic hyperdense collection in perisplenic region on plain CT indicating a subcapsular hematoma (Fig. 1A). The subcapsular hematoma is 2 cm in thickness. Contrast enhanced CT (Fig. 1B) shows an irregular nonenhancing area in the superior part of spleen extending from posterior to anterior aspect indicating the splenic laceration. It is 3 cm deep from the capsule. Splenic CT injury grading scale is GRADE II. In this case subcapsular hematoma was also seen around the liver (Fig. 1C). Surgical emphysema is seen in left lateral abdominal wall and fracture is seen in left 8th rib (Fig. 1D).

Comments and Explanation

The major CT features of blunt splenic injuries are lacerations, subcapsular and parenchymal hematomas, active hemorrhage, hemoperitoneum and vascular injury. CT scanning can also provide an accurate appraisal of coexisting abdominal injuries, such as injuries to the retroperitoneum, abdominal wall, and can exclude the presence of lesions requiring surgery, such as bowel or pancreatic injuries.

Opinion

Splenic laceration with splenic subcapsular hematoma, subcapsular hepatic hematoma, surgical emphysema and rib fracture.

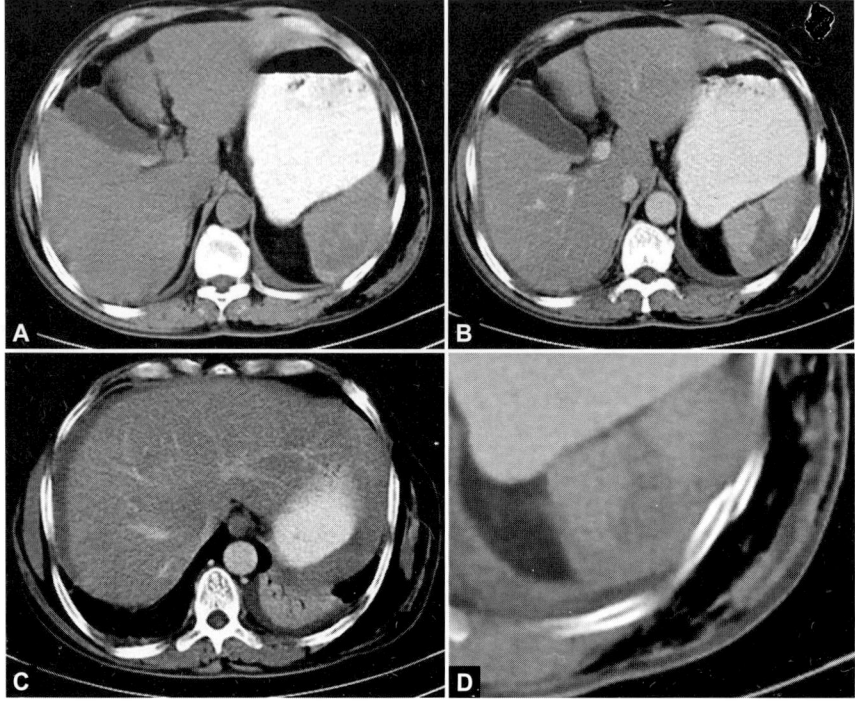

Figs 1A to D

Clinical Discussion

Spleen is the most frequently injured solid organ in blunt trauma to the abdomen. Splenic injury is often associated with left rib fractures and other organ injuries like kidney. CT is highly accurate in diagnosing splenic injury. Splenic parenchyma should be assessed in portal venous phase as the heterogeneous contrast-enhancement seen on arterial phase can mimic splenic laceration/contusion. Arterial phase scanning is useful in assessing vascular injuries such as pseudoaneurysm and AV fistula. CT scan findings that indicate splenic injury include hemoperitoneum, subcapsular hematoma and laceration, active bleeding and contained vascular injuries including arteriovenous fistula and pseudoaneurysm. Hemoperitoneum refers to localized fluid collections around the spleen with an elevated Hounsfield unit. Briskly bleeding splenic lacerations may show blood density fluid throughout the abdomen. Subcapsular hematoma is seen as a crescentic low attenuation area along the lateral margin which flattens the normal convex margin of spleen. Intrasplenic hematoma is seen as round to oval hypodense area. Linear hypodense area represents laceration. Contrast blush or extravasation is defined as hyperdense areas within the splenic parenchyma that represent traumatic disruption or pseudoaneurysm of the splenic vasculature. Active extravasation of contrast implies ongoing bleeding and need for urgent intervention.

Splenic CT Injury Grading Scale

- GRADE I: Laceration < 1 cm deep, subcapsular hematoma < 1 cm diameter
- GRADE II: Laceration 1–3 cm deep, subcapsular hematoma 1–3 cm diameter
- GRADE III: Laceration >3 cm deep, subcapsular hematoma >3 cm diameter, parenchymal hematoma > 5 cm
- GRADE IV: Laceration involving segmental or hilar vessels, producing major devascularization (> 25% of spleen)
- GRADE V: Shattered spleen or avulsed spleen with total devascularization.

CASE 53

Splenic Abscess

CASE

A 48-year-old female with history of pyrexia of unknown origin subjected to CT abdomen and pelvis.

Radiological Findings on CT Examination

CT abdomen, coronal reconstruction shows splenomegaly (Fig. 1). There is a well defined hypodense lesion with a thick peripherally enhancing wall and mild perilesional edema in the upper pole of spleen suggestive of splenic abscess.

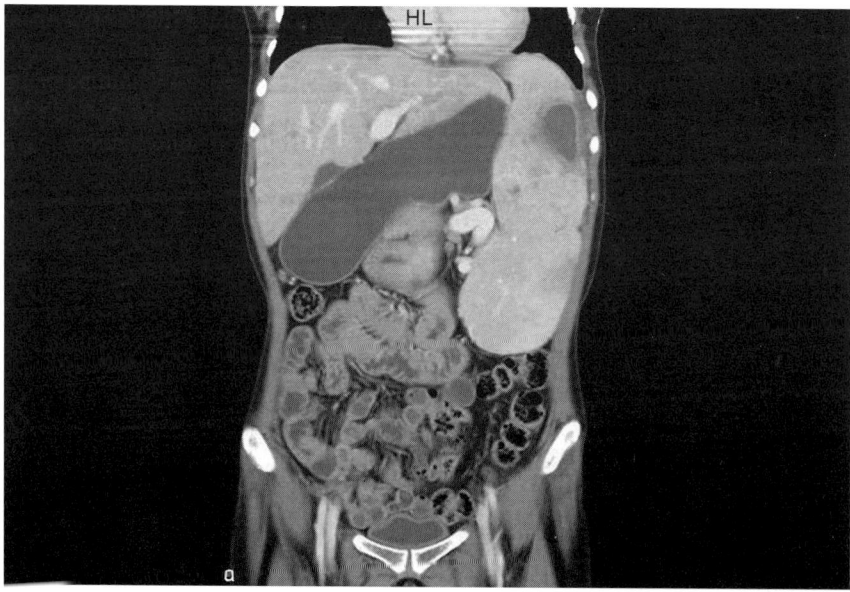

Fig. 1

Comments and Explanation

Abscesses are localized collections of necrotic inflammatory tissue caused by bacterial, parasitic or fungal agents. Ultrasonography abdomen shows hypoechoic to heteroechoic collection with or without internal septae and air. CT shows low attenuation, ill defined lesion with peripheral contrast enhancement. It may rarely contain gas bubbles or air fluid level. MR imaging shows abscess as a fluid intensity, low intensity on T1WI and high intensity on T2WI.

Opinion

Splenic abscess.

Clinical Discussion

Abscess of the spleen is a rather rare clinical entity. Patients with recognized risk factors are immunocompromised, endocarditis, diabetes mellitus, immunosuppression, trauma, drug abuse. They are more frequently detected in middle-aged and older individuals, with no obvious preference for either sex. The clinical manifestations of splenic abscesses usually include abdominal pain, exclusively located or, at least, more intensely described in the upper-left-quadrant area. Fever, nausea, vomiting and anorexia may be also present in various combinations. Laboratory findings are consistent with the acute phase of infection, but their exact nature is determined by the pathogen isolated from the abscess. The most common pathogens detected include *Staphylococcus* and *Streptococcus*. Due to the seriousness of the potential implications, including a threat to life itself, the most usual treatment currently applied is splenectomy, which is followed by rapid clinical improvement. Percutaneus imaging guided drainage is minimally invasive procedure.

SECTION 13

Vascular

54. Superior Mesenteric Artery Syndrome
55. Superior Mesenteric Artery Thrombosis
56. Accessory Renal Artery Stenosis
57. Aneurysm of Abdominal Aorta
58. Inferior Vena Cava Thrombus
59. Aortic Thrombus
60. Portal Vein Thrombosis

CASE 54

Superior Mesenteric Artery Syndrome

CASE

A 15-year-old female presented to the department of radiology with pain in epigastric region and nausea since 2–3 months.

Radiological Findings on CT Examination

Axial and sagittal reconstructed images of contrast enhanced CT abdomen shows reduced distance between aorta and superior mesenteric artery (SMA) and also there is evidence of reduced angle between the aorta and SMA (Figs 1A to D).

Comments and Explanation

Superior mesenteric artery syndrome is a condition in which the distance between the aorta and SMA and the angle between them is reduced which leads to the extrinsic vascular compression of third portion of duodenum and the patient presents with abdominal cramps and repeated vomiting.

Opinion

Superior mesenteric artery syndrome.

Clinical Discussion

The superior mesenteric artery syndrome occurs in older children and adolescents. Commonly females are affected by this. Transverse duodenum courses caudal to the SMA origin, which normally forms an angle of 45° with the aorta. Any factor which narrows the aortomesenteric angle to approximately 10–22° can compress the transverse duodenum, resulting in SMA syndrome. Causes include weight loss, prolonged bed rest in the supine position, corrective surgery for scoliosis, and congenital causes (high insertion of the duodenum at the ligament of Treitz or low origin of the SMA). The patient often presents with chronic upper abdominal symptoms such as epigastric pain, nausea, voluminous

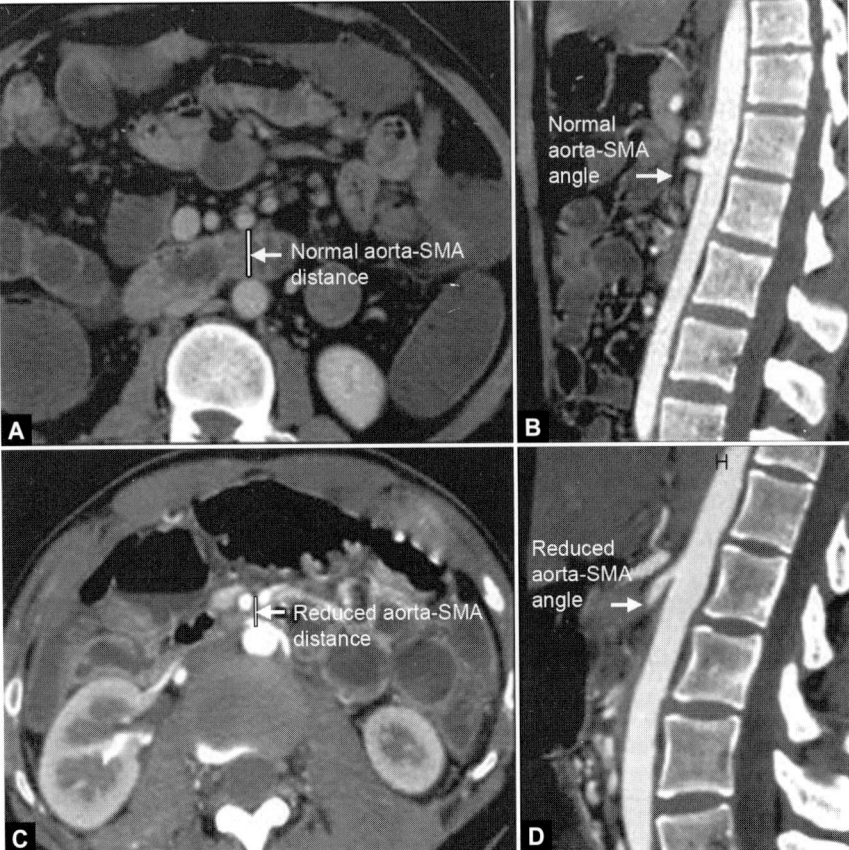

Figs 1A to D

vomiting (bilious or partially digested food), postprandial discomfort, early satiety, and sometimes, subacute small bowel obstruction. Diagnosis requires clinical and imaging correlation. Diagnostic imaging studies include CT, fluoroscopic upper GI studies, and abdominal ultrasound. Fluoroscopy is particularly useful, providing real-time imaging during contrast transit. This will show dilation of the first and second portions of the duodenum as it passes anterior to the aorta. A partial or complete obstruction to flow may be present. There is often hyperperistalsis in the proximal segments of duodenum. CT criteria for the diagnosis of superior mesenteric artery syndrome include an aortomesenteric angle of less than 22° and an aortomesenteric distance of less than 8–10 mm. CT scan will show pronounced dilatation of the stomach and proximal duodenum with vertical linear compression defect in the transverse duodenum, overlying the spine, and abrupt caliber change distal to the compression defect. Initial treatment is typically conservative and includes adequate nutrition, nasogastric decompression, and proper positioning after eating. Enteral feeding via feeding tube passed distal to the point of obstruction is often required. Surgery is indicated when conservative measures are ineffective.

CASE 55

Superior Mesenteric Artery Thrombosis

CASE

A 55-year-old female presented to the department of radiology with acute pain in abdomen.

Radiological Findings on CT Examination

Contrast enhanced axial and sagittal CT images of abdomen show wall thickening and eccentric thrombosis of superior mesenteric artery (Figs 1A and B).

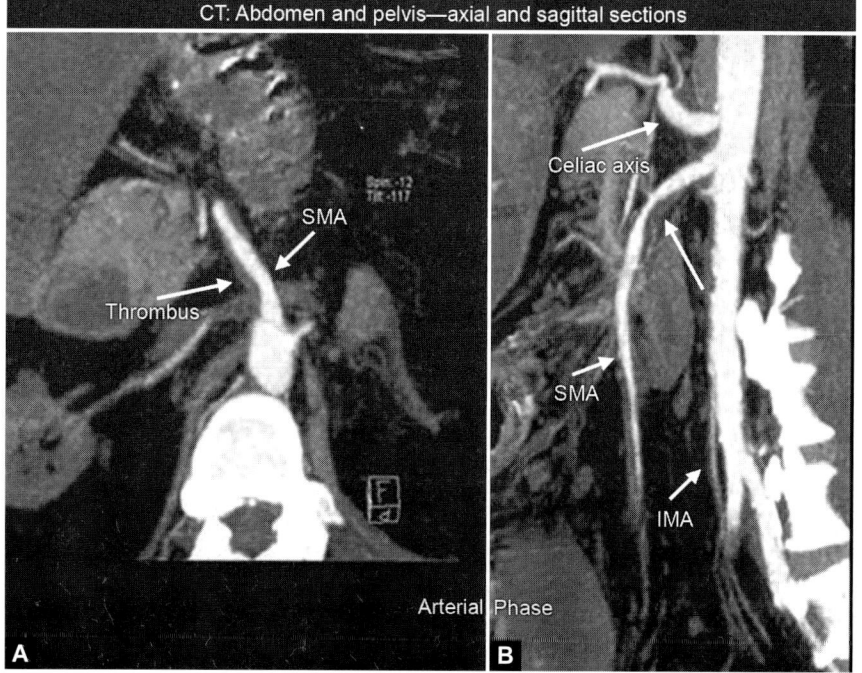

Figs 1A and B

In Other Cases

- Contrast enhanced CT abdomen shows complete occlusion of the SMA lumen by thrombus seen just after its origin from abdominal aorta (Figs 2A and B).
- CT mesenteric angiography shows thrombus in proximal part of SMA starting from its origin from abdominal aorta. The distal SMA is patent (Figs 3A and B).

Comments and Explanation

Thrombosis of the superior mesenteric artery is most often associated with a pre-existing atherosclerotic lesion that already compromises flow. The most common pre-existing pathology found in patients with acute mesenteric thrombosis is atherosclerosis. The atherosclerotic plaque, usually at the origin of the SMA, grows over time. The SMA is the most common visceral branch to thrombose. Complete block of superior mesenteric artery leads to necrosis of bowel, perforation and then peritonitis with fatal consequences. CT angiography is important for diagnosis and it shows complete nonvisualization of SMA. Also it can depict the bowel viability and diagnose complications like perforation and peritonitis. Findings on CT scan in acute SMA occlusion include lack of enhancement of the lumen of SMA and its branches. Other findings which can be seen in thrombosis are mesenteric fat stranding due to mesenteric ischemia. Intense mucosal enhancement of bowel wall with thickening, bowel distension with intraluminal fluid accumulation, portal venous gas, free fluid and free intra-abdominal air.

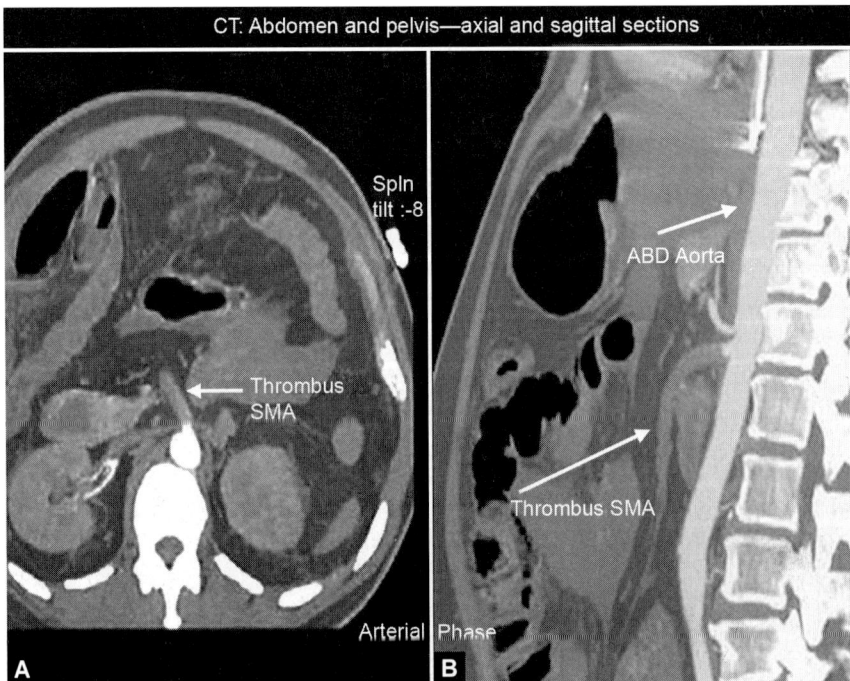

Figs 2A and B

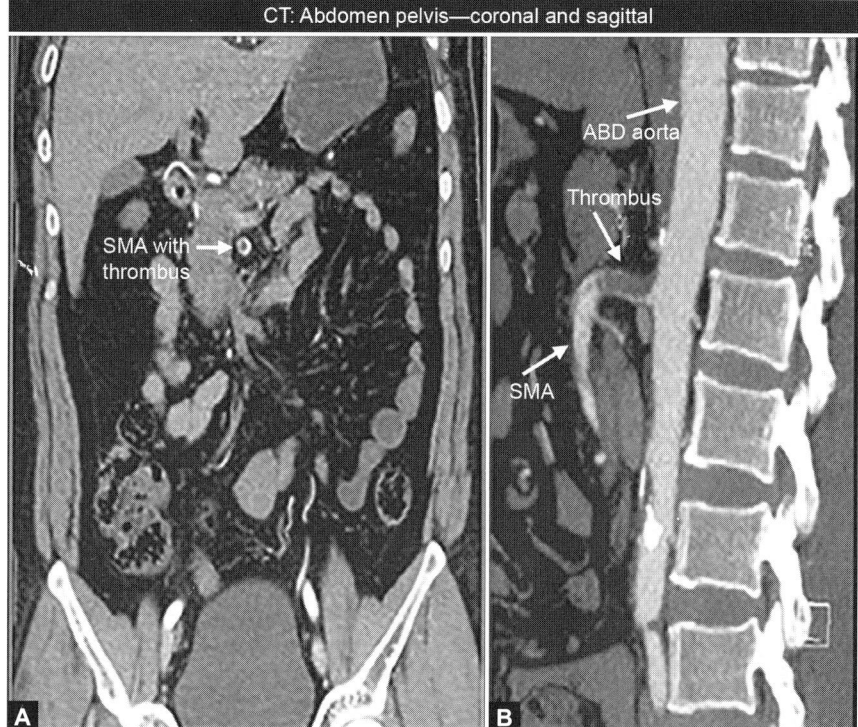

Figs 3A and B

Opinion

Superior mesenteric artery thrombosis.

Clinical Discussion

Patients with acute mesenteric artery thrombosis present with a long history of weight loss, postprandial pain. Symptoms worsen over time. Patients complain of severe, acute, unrelenting abdominal pain. They may also complain of frank blood in their stools. Medical history may be significant for stroke, MI, or peripheral artery disease. Patients may have a long history of smoking or uncontrolled diabetes. Clinical presentation is variable and depends upon the extent of luminal narrowing. A mesenteric arterial embolism results in a different extension of the infarcted areas because the emboli can occlude the vessel tree to different levels. The poor prognosis of patients with mesenteric arterial occlusions is most likely due to the proximal location of the occlusion in the vessel tree; this determines a more extensive bowel infarction and the need for extended intestinal resection. The prerequisite for success of a revascularization is prompt diagnosis.

CASE 56

Accessory Renal Artery Stenosis

CASE

A 53-year-old male patient with history of hypertension presented for renal angiogram to the department of radiology to rule out renal artery stenosis.

Radiological Findings on CT Examination

CT renal angiography (Fig. 1) reveals normal main renal arteries, an accessory renal artery is present, and it has a right lateral origin from the aorta proximal to the bifurcation which shows stenosis at its origin (arrow).

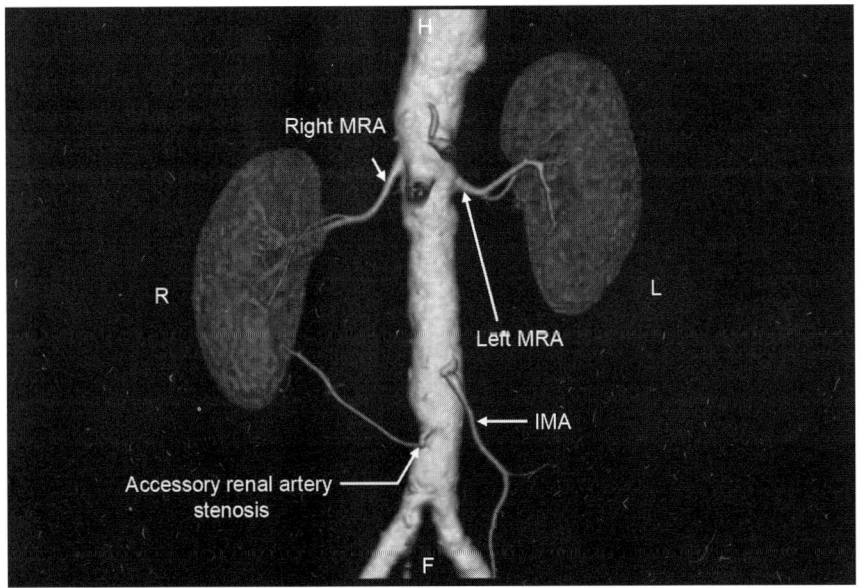

Fig. 1 *(For color version, see plate 3)*

Comments and Explanation

Accessory renal arteries are a common variant and are present in 25% of the population. Most commonly accessory renal arteries arise from the abdominal aorta and supply to the inferior pole of the kidney although they can rarely arise from celiac trunk, mesenteric arteries or other abdominal arteries.

Opinion

Accessory renal artery stenosis.

Clinical Discussion

CT angiography with MIP and quantitative measurement of stenosis is an accurate noninvasive technique in the diagnosis of renal artery stenosis. Accessory renal arteries are reliably identified by means of CTA. CT can detect stenosis in the mainstem artery or its intrarenal branches, with a high degree of accuracy. It is an important pathological sign that radiologist has to evaluate and assess because of its association with hypertension. Multidetector computed tomographic angiography (MDCTA) help to correctly evaluate accessory renal arteries in addition to renal arteries. Not all accessory renal artery stenosis are associated with renovascular hypertension. In this case considering the age of the patient it is less likely to be associated with hypertension as it is more likely to be essential hypertension.

CASE 57

Aneurysm of Abdominal Aorta

CASE

A 62-year-old male with intermittent claudication since one month and vague abdominal pain in supine position relieved in lateral position, was subjected to CT angiogram (abdomen and pelvis).

Radiological Findings on CT Examination

3D volume rendered images (Figs 1A and B) of CT angiogram shows focal aneurysm; pedicle is seen to arise from the anterior aspect, just above the bifurcation of abdominal aorta.

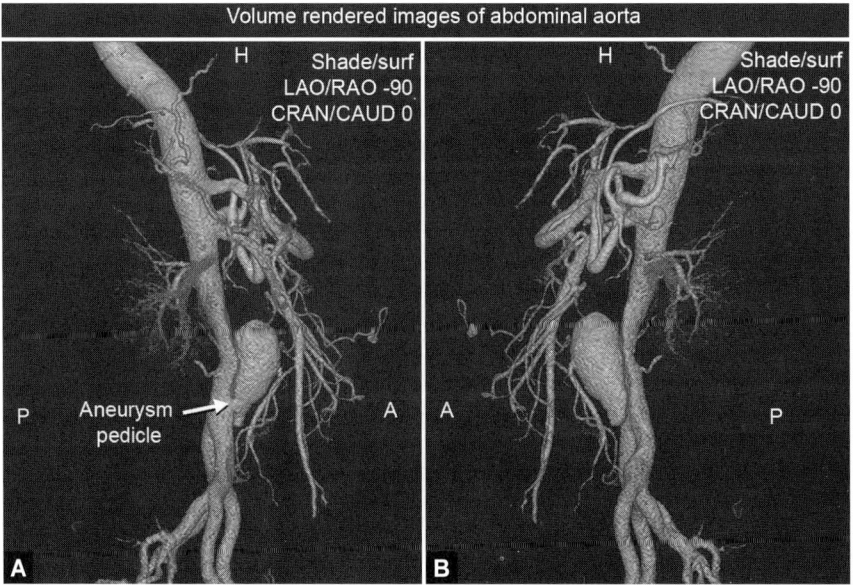

Figs 1A and B *(For color version, see plate 4)*

Comments and Explanation

An **abdominal aortic aneurysm (AAA)** is defined as focal dilatation of the abdominal aorta that is 50% greater than the proximal normal segment or that is greater than 3 cm in maximum diameter. Majority of abdominal aortic aneurysms originate below the renal arteries and can extend to involve the aortic bifurcation and proximal iliac arteries. AAA's are frequently asymptomatic and discovered during radiologic or physical examinations performed for other reasons. Approximately 50% of abdominal aortic aneurysms are visible on a plain radiograph of the lateral lumbar spine due to calcification within its wall. Ultrasound is noninvasive modality and provides accurate measurement of the diameter of aorta, and can discern free intraperitoneal blood. Unfortunately, US is not particularly helpful for assessment of aneurysmal rupture, nor it is useful for imaging the thoracic or suprarenal aorta, because of interference from overlying lung. CT scan accurately demonstrates dilation of the aorta and involvement of major branch vessels proximally and distally. This information helps in determining the appropriate intervention, which may be either surgical or endovascular repair. "Crescent sign" i.e. peripheral high-attenuating crescent in aneurysm wall, i.e. acute intramural hematoma is a sign of impending rupture. CT also shows the other organs in the abdomen and demonstrates involvement or displacement of organs. The location and number of the renal arteries, caliber of the aneurysm, degree of calcification, lengths of the neck, iliac artery, and presence of mural thrombus are readily assessed. CT angiography (CTA) allows multiplanar assessment of the aneurysm and associated relevant vessels. CT is also helpful in detecting complications like aneurysm rupture and dissection. CT scan findings in case of aneurysm rupture include anterior displacement of kidney, extravasation of contrast material, fluid collection/hematoma within posterior pararenal and perirenal spaces, free intraperitoneal fluid.

Opinion

Aneurysm of abdominal aorta.

Clinical Discussion

Normal size of abdominal aorta >50 years of age is about 2 cm. Prevalence of abdominal aortic aneurysm increases with age, atherosclerotic disease and white race. Risk factors include male gender, age >75 years, prior vascular disease, hypertension, cigarette smoking, family history and hypercholesterolemia. Clinically most of the patients are asymptomatic but may complain of abdominal mass and pain. When the triad of abdominal or flank pain, shock, and a pulsatile abdominal mass are present, the diagnosis of ruptured AAA is relatively straightforward. Abdominal aneurysms are complicated by rupture, distal thromboembolism, infection, spontaneous occlusion of aorta. Patients with AAA < 4 cm will need serial ultrasound evaluations every 6 months. If growth exceeds 0.5 cm in six months, the aneurysm becomes > 4 cm, symptoms related to the aneurysm are present, or a complicated aneurysm is present, surgical repair is usually indicated.

CASE 58

Inferior Vena Cava Thrombus

CASE

A 43-year-old male patient presented with bilateral pedal edema and was referred to radiology department for CT abdomen.

Radiological Findings on CT Scan

CT scan abdomen (Fig. 1) shows a large intraluminal filling defect in the entire length of inferior vena cava (IVC) extending into both common iliac veins. Few collateral vessels are seen in this reconstruction. Superior vena cava (SVC) and pulmonary vessels are normal.

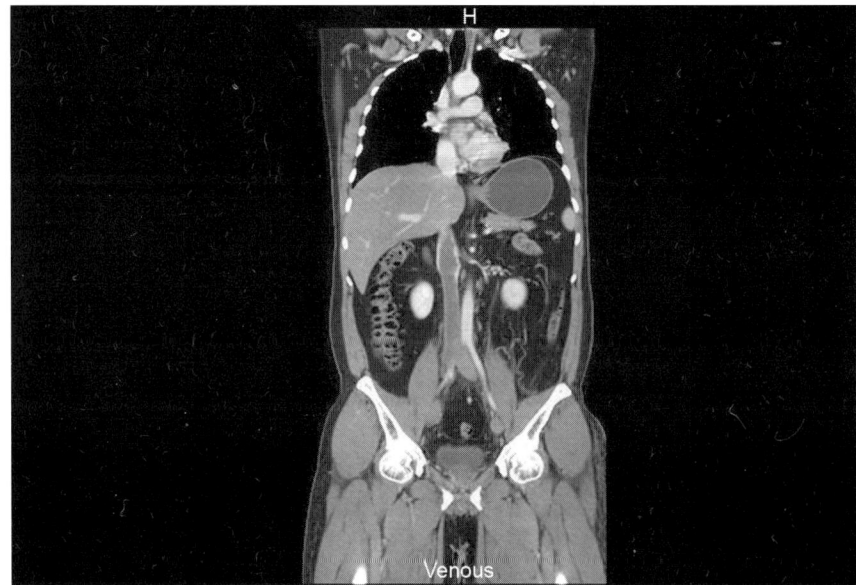

Fig. 1

Comments and Explanation

The most reliable, noninvasive method to establish a diagnosis of IVC anomalies is CT scan with intravenous (IV) contrast or MRI. CT scan is a good imaging modality for evaluating the retroperitoneal space. Another accurate, but more invasive, imaging modality is venography, which is particularly useful if any surgery is planned. A bland thrombus results from external compression of the IVC by a neoplastic lesion, so the IVC is usually narrowed at the site of thrombosis. In contrast, tumor thrombus expands the IVC. Tumor thrombus will often show continuity with primary tumor. In arterial phase, neovascularity may be appreciated in tumor thrombus.

Opinion

IVC thrombosis.

Clinical Discussion

Inferior vena cava thrombosis is an essential diagnosis while evaluating any neoplastic lesion, or portal hypertension. Etiology includes hypercoagulable state, IVC filters, catheters, extension from tumors like renal cell carcinoma, leiomyosarcoma of IVC. The classic presentation of IVC thrombosis includes bilateral lower extremity edema with dilated, visible superficial abdominal veins. In addition, if the thrombus is confined to the cava and does not involve the iliac or femoral system, the collateral pathways form along the posterior abdominal wall. This scenario may have significant impact on surgical procedures involving this anatomic region. Thrombosis occurring at the level of the renal veins raises the possibility of renal cell carcinoma. Patient can present with bilateral pedal edema or pulmonary embolism. Any neoplastic lesion can cause IVC thrombosis, renal cell carcinoma is the most common malignancy to extend into IVC. Other tumors that have a tendency for IVC thrombosis are hepatocellular carcinoma and Wilms' tumor.

CASE 59

Aortic Thrombus

CASE

A 55-year-old male with complaint of pain in abdomen since three days was subjected to CT abdomen and pelvis.

Findings on CT Examination

CT aortography shows acute long segment thrombotic occlusion of infra-renal abdominal aorta extending to bilateral common iliac arteries (Figs 1A, B and E). Short segment occlusion of inferior mesenteric artery is seen (Fig. 1D). Bilateral main renal arteries are normal in their course and calibre (Fig. 1C).

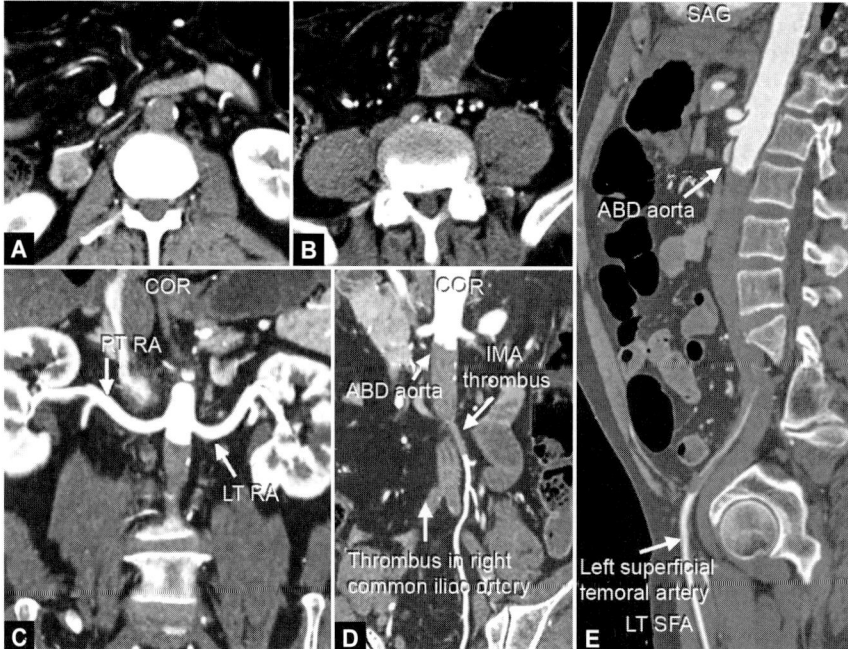

Figs 1A to E

Comments and Explanation

Transabdominal USG allows for detailed depiction of intraluminal thrombus (ILT) morphology. With the use of low-frequency (e.g. 4-MHz) probes, the echogenic ILT will be delineated against the echo-free aortic lumen. USG can show calcifications in the ILT as areas of hyperechogenicity accompanied by an echo-free shadow artifact. Contrast-enhanced CT allows for a detailed depiction of ILT morphology by delineating the low-attenuating ILT against the contrast filled, high-attenuating aortic lumen. With contrast-enhanced CT, a halo-shaped area of high attenuation in the thrombus—the "Crescent sign" can be visualized. CT shows calcifications in the intraluminal thrombus better than any other imaging method.

Opinion

Infrarenal aortic thrombus extending to bilateral common iliac and inferior mesenteric artery.

Clinical Discussion

Atheromatous occlusion of the distal abdominal aorta at the bifurcation into the common iliac arteries is called Leriche syndrome. Triad of symptoms includes claudication in the legs or buttocks absent or diminished femoral pulses, erectile dysfunction. Usually affects younger males 30–40 years of age. Risk factors include cigarette smoking, hypercholesterolemia and diabetes. Development of the disease is slow and collaterals develop, limb-threatening ischemic disease does not tend to occur. Treatment options include aortoiliac bypass surgery or kissing balloon angioplasty and stent implantation.

CASE 60

Portal Vein Thrombosis

CASE

A 30-year-old female with history of pain in abdomen, nausea and vomiting since 5 days was referred to the department of radiology for CT abdomen.

Radiological Findings on CT Examination

Contrast enhanced CT abdomen reveals failure of opacification following IV contrast of main portal vein and splenic vein (Fig. 1A arrows), portal confluence (Fig. 1B arrow) and superior mesenteric vein (Fig. 1C arrow). This is thrombosis of portal vein, splenic vein and superior mesenteric vein with resultant differential enhancement in right lobe of liver (Fig. 1D).

In another case of contrast enhanced CT abdomen there is failure of opacification of left branch of portal vein because of thrombosis (Figs 2A and B arrow). Multiple calculi are also seen in gallbladder (Fig. 2B).

Comments and Explanation

The thrombus is observed as an echogenic lesion within the portal vein, though a recently formed thrombus may be anechoic and is not seen on standard gray-scale ultrasound. Contrast-enhanced CT scan has the advantage over ultrasound in displaying varices and parenchymal hepatic abnormalities. Portal venous phase of CT shows partial or complete nonopacification of portal vein or its branches. MRI is helpful if hepatic parenchymal detail is required. MRI can also quantitate portal and hepatic vessel flow, which is required in the planning of interventions, such as shunt surgery, transjugular intrahepatic portosystemic shunt (TIPS) or liver transplantation. Acute clot (< 5 weeks) appears hyperintense on both T1- and T2-weighted images, whereas older clots appear hyperintense only on T2-weighted images. Tumor thrombi can be differentiated from bland thrombi because they appear more hyperintense on T2-weighted images and enhance with contrast. Cavernous transformation of portal vein is a sequelae of portal vein thrombosis and is replacement of portal vein by multiple venous channels. This develops in patients whose portal vein does not recanalize or

Case 60: Portal Vein Thrombosis

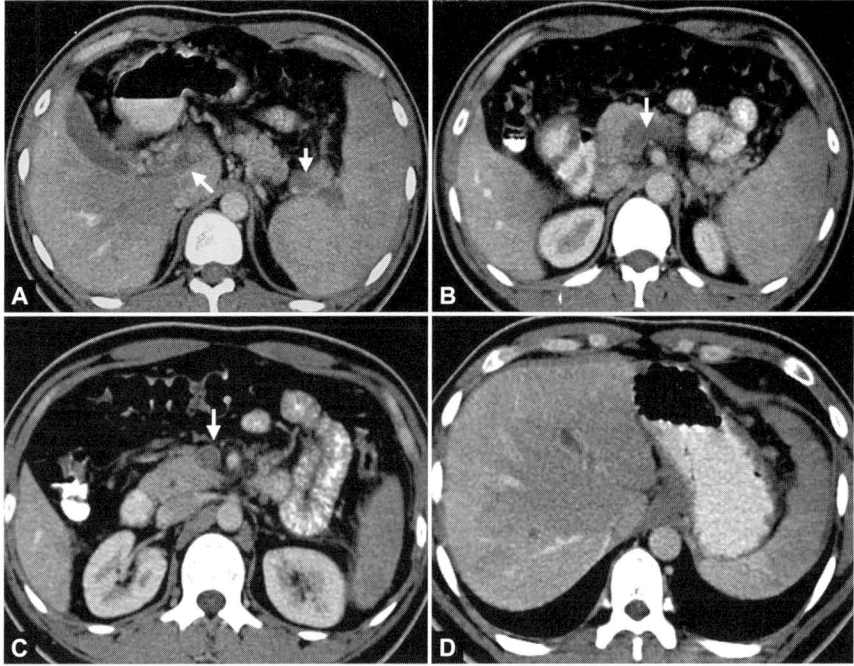

Figs 1A to D

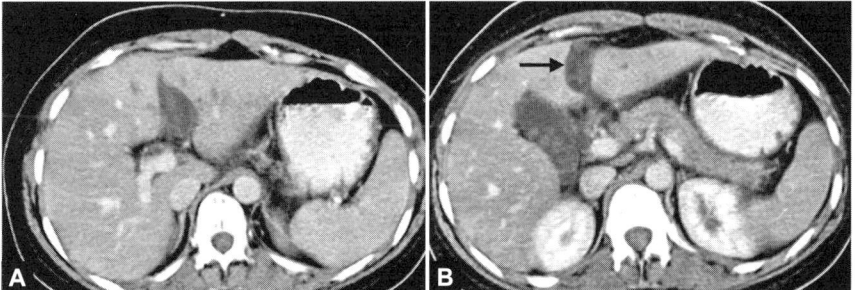

Figs 2A and B

only partially re-canalises collateral veins dilate and become serpiginous. On USG cavernous transformation appears as numerous tortuous vessels occupying the portal vein bed. Triphasic CT can confirm the diagnosis by demonstrating numerous vascular channels in the region of portal vein which enhance during portal phase and not during arterial phase distinguishing it from arteriovenous malformation.

Opinion

Portal vein thrombosis.

Clinical Discussion

Portal vein thrombosis is rare and clinically may be asymptomatic. Thrombus may be acute or chronic. Local factors favoring or precipitating development of portal vein thrombosis include local inflammatory lesions, neonatal omphalitis, diverticulitis, appendicitis, pancreatitis, duodenal ulcer, cholecystitis, tuberculous lymphadenitis, injury to the portal venous system, surgical portacaval shunting, splenectomy, colectomy, gastrectomy, cancer of abdominal organs and cirrhosis. Symptoms often presents as gastrointestinal bleeding, variceal bleeding, ascites, and abdominal pain. Portal hypertension and mesenteric ischemia are complications of portal vein thrombosis. Treatment options include systemic anticoagulation, endovascular infusion of thrombolytic agents: percutaneous transhepatic approach and surgical thrombectomy.

SECTION 14

Adrenal

61. Adrenal Adenoma
62. Pheochromocytoma
63. Adrenal Metastases

CASE 61

Adrenal Adenoma

CASE

A 50-year-old male referred to the department of radiology with vague dull abdominal pain in left hypochondriac region for CT abdomen.

Radiological Findings on CT Examination

Pre and post contrast axial images of abdomen (Figs 1A and B) show normal right adrenal gland. Left adrenal gland shows a nonenhancing, solid, well-defined iso to hyperdense lesion, suggestive of left adrenal adenoma with no evidence of fat stranding or infiltration of surrounding tissues.

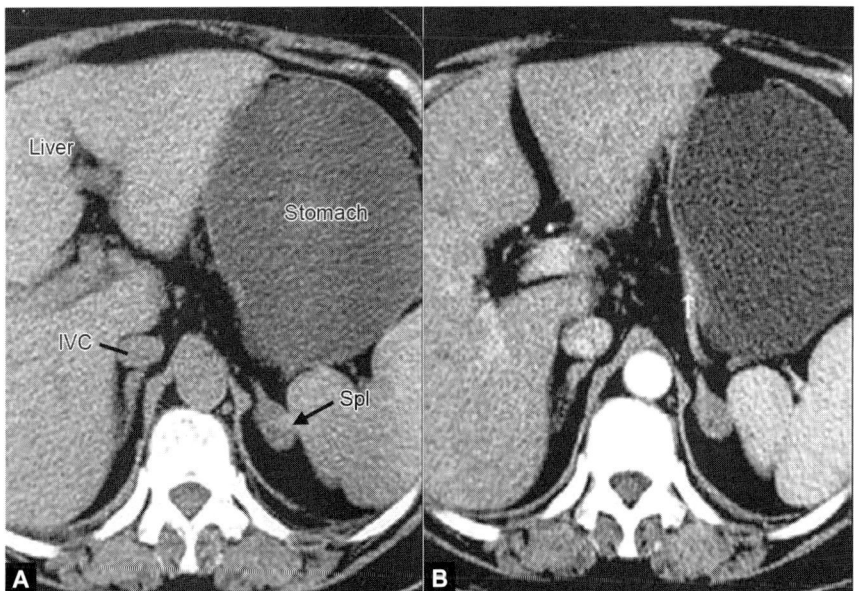

Figs 1A and B

Comments and Explanation

The majority of adrenal adenomas are nonfunctioning; in such cases patients are asymptomatic. Patients with hyper functioning adrenal gland adenomas present with manifestations of excess hormone secretion, such as Cushing's syndrome due to excess cortisol production, Conn's syndrome (due to excess aldosterone production) or sex-hormone related symptoms. Adenomas can be divided into those that have typical or atypical appearances. Typical adenomas are small, less than 3 cm and are of low density. They show homogeneous appearance. Atypical adenomas are large, more than 3 cm and show hemorrhage, calcification, necrosis and absence of fat. If greater than 6 cm chances of it being malignant is 85%. CT is a well established modality for investigating adrenal masses and uses the fact that the majority of adenomas have high lipid content. Noncontrast CT is performed and the CT number (Hounsfield units (HU)) of the mass is measured. If the CT value is ≤10 HU it is considered to be a benign adenoma on the basis of its fat content. If the CT value is >10 HU, enhanced 60 seconds and a 15 minutes delayed postcontrast CT are obtained, and the enhancement washout is calculated. The percentage of absolute enhancement washout can be thus calculated:

$$\% \text{ washout} = \frac{\text{enhanced attenuation value} - \text{delayed attenuation value}}{\text{enhanced attenuation value} - \text{nonenhanced attenuation value}} \times 100$$

The enhanced attenuation value is the attenuation value of the mass in HU, 60 seconds after contrast administration. The delayed attenuation value is the attenuation value of the mass in HU, 10–15 minutes after contrast administration.

If the enhancement washout is >50%, the diagnosis of a benign lipid poor adenoma is made. If the washout is <50%, the mass is considered indeterminate, and a biopsy may be necessary to make a diagnosis. Metastatic deposits are usually larger and more heterogeneous than adenomas and do not have intracellular fat. Frequently in clinical practice, only postcontrast images are available. In these patients, the percentage 'relative' enhancement washout can be thus calculated:

$$\% \text{ relative washout} = \frac{\text{enhanced attenuation value} - \text{delayed attenuation value}}{\text{enhanced attenuation value}} \times 100$$

At 15 minutes, if a relative enhancement washout of 40% or higher is achieved, this has a sensitivity of 96–100% and a specificity of 100% for the diagnosis of an adenoma. Therefore a combination of unenhanced CT and enhancement washout characteristics correctly separates most adrenal masses as adenomas or metastases. Adrenal cortical adenoma is a common benign tumor arising from the cortex of the adrenal gland. It commonly occurs in adults, but it can be found in persons of any age. Adenomas typically demonstrate rapid washout, which is defined as an absolute percentage washout (APW) of more than 60% and a relative percentage washout (RPW) of more than 40% on delayed images. The majority of lesions are nonfunctioning. Although CT does not allow differentiation of functioning from nonfunctioning masses, the presence of contralateral adrenal atrophy suggests that a lesion may be functioning, because pituitary adrenocorticotropic hormone secretion is suppressed by elevated cortisol levels.

Opinion

Adrenal adenoma.

Clinical Discussion

Nonfunctioning adrenal adenomas are asymptomatic. However the functioning adrenal adenoma presents with pheochromocytoma like symptoms which include episodic attacks, palpitations, sweating, headaches, and abdominal pain, as well as labile hypertension. Vital signs may include findings of hypertension, postural hypotension, and tachycardia. Hypertensive retinopathy is present. Skin findings present as hirsutism. General signs include central obesity and gynecomastia. Adrenal adenoma can be diagnosed using chemical shift MRI. The characterization of a lesion as an adenoma relies on the ratio of a decreased relative signal intensity from in phase to opposed phase images and the ratio of adrenal mass and various organs on T2-weighted and chemical shift images. Small adrenal mass with manifestations of hormonal excess need resection, as do large (> 3 to 5 cm) nonfunctioning adrenal mass lesions as they are considered potentially malignant.

CASE 62

Pheochromocytoma

CASE

A 14-year-old hypertensive male child with complaints of giddiness was subjected to CT abdomen and pelvis.

Radiological Finding on CT Examination

CT abdomen shows a well defined round, hypodense lesion seen superior to the left renal hilum (Figs 1A to C), the lesion shows heterogeneous enhancement and is seen separate from left kidney, pancreas and left renal vessel.

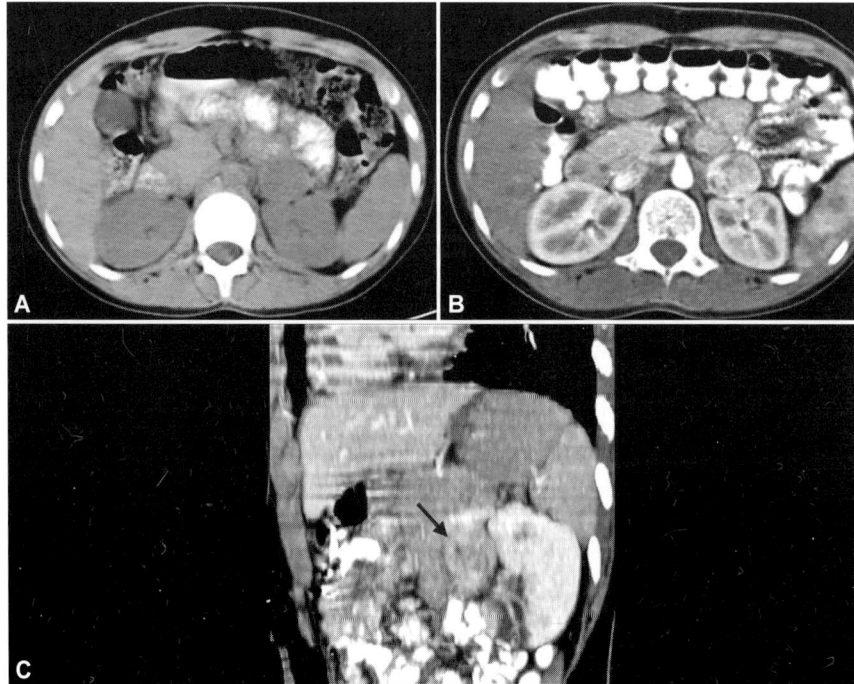

Figs 1A to C

Comments and Explanation

Adrenal tumors tend to be large at presentation. On CT examination lesions have a precontrast attenuation >10 HU. Most lesions vigorously enhance (>80 HU) and have less than 60% washout of contrast on delayed images. There may be areas of necrosis and cystic change. Up to 7% demonstrate areas of calcification. On T1WI pheochromocytoma appears slightly hypointense to the remainder of the adrenal and appears heterogeneous if necrotic or hemorrhagic. On T2WI it appears hyperintense (lighted bulb sign) and enhances heterogeneously. MRI is preferred for detection of extra-adrenal pheochromocytoma. Differential diagnosis includes adrenal adenomas, adrenal carcinomas and adrenal metastases.

Opinion

Adrenal pheochromocytoma.

Clinical Discussion

Pheochromocytomas are rare, catecholamine secreting, neuroendocrine tumor usually found in medulla of the adrenal gland originating in the chromaffin cells. Extra-adrenal tumors are called paraganglioneuromas. Most pheochromocytomas produce epinephrine and norepinephrine. Sometimes dopamine is secreted. About 10% tumors are malignant and occur at any age with peak in 3rd to 5th decades, with no sex predilection.

Locations of extra adrenal pheochromocytomas include the organ of Zuckerkandl which is close to the origin of the inferior mesenteric artery, bladder wall, heart, mediastinum, and carotid and glomus jugulare bodies. Patients complain of headache, palpitations and diaphoresis with hypertension, weakness, nausea, tremors, anxiety and weight loss. Pheochromocytomas are associated with von Hippel-Lindau disease, neurofibromatosis, multiple endocrine neoplasia (MEN) 2A (Sipple syndrome) and 2B, tuberous sclerosis, Sturge-Weber syndrome. Plasma metanephrine and urine catecholamine, creatinine, vanilmandelic acid and metanephrine levels after 24 hours are useful for diagnosis. Resection of tumor is a treatment of choice.

CASE 63

Adrenal Metastases

CASE

A 55-year-old female with complaints of cough and breathlessness was subjected to high-resolution computed tomography (HRCT) chest.

Radiological Findings on CT Examination

Large enhancing lobulated mass lesion seen in right upper lobe in paratracheal region with nonenhancing necrotic areas. The lesion closely abuts the right main bronchus, upper lobe bronchus, superior vena cava and extends to precarinal region with loss of fat planes. These findings are suggestive of bronchogenic carcinoma (Fig. 1A). Multiple small rounded metastatic nodules seen in bilateral lungs (Fig. 1B). A well defined lobulated peripherally enhancing soft tissue density lesion in left adrenal gland is suggestive of adrenal metastases (Fig. 1C).

Comments and Explanation

Primary tumors that metastasize to the adrenal glands are lung carcinoma, colorectal carcinoma, breast carcinoma, pancreatic carcinoma, renal cell carcinoma, hepatocellular carcinoma, malignant melanoma. CT is the investigation of choice for evaluation of adrenal metastasis and most of the lesions show percentage enhancement of washout, similar to that of lipid-poor adrenal adenoma. On MR it appears as T1 hypointense and T2 hyperintense lesion and shows progressive enhancement on post contrast scan. A diagnosis of adrenal metastasis is important in examining patients with cancer because the metastasis indicates inoperable stage IV disease (except in ipsilateral renal cancer). Adrenal metastases have no specific imaging features. Statistically most nonadenomas are metastases.

Opinion

Primary lung carcinoma with pulmonary and adrenal metastasis.

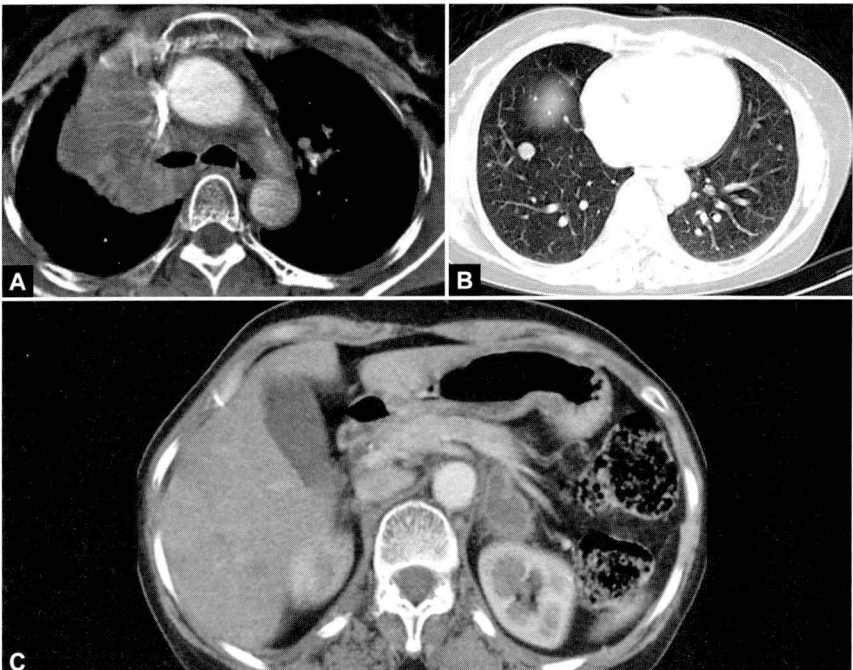

Figs 1A to C

Clinical Discussion

A patient may develop symptoms related to insufficient production of steroid hormones by the involved adrenal glands (adrenal insufficiency or Addisonian state). Adrenal insufficiency is characterized by weakness, low blood pressure, low blood sugar, low blood sodium and high potassium levels, and darkening of the skin. The most effective treatment for adrenal metastases is to treat the primary cancer, usually with chemotherapy and/or radiation therapy. If adrenal insufficiency is present, then steroid hormone replacement should be given. For patients in whom the adrenal is the only site of metastatic disease and the primary cancer is well controlled, the adrenal metastasis may be treated by either radiation therapy or surgical removal. In these cases, adrenalectomy can often be done using minimally invasive technique.

SECTION 15

Renal

64. Renal Aplasia
65. Dysplastic Kidney
66. Polycystic Kidneys
67. Pelviureteric Junction Obstruction
68. Obstructive Uropathy
69. Emphysematous Pyelonephritis
70. Renal Vein Thrombosis
71. Renal Laceration
72. Renal Angiomyolipoma
73. Wilms' Tumor
74. Renal Cell Carcinoma

CASE 64

Renal Aplasia

CASE

A 35-year-old male presented to the department of radiology as part of routine health check up.

Radiological Findings on CT Examination

Axial post contrast CT image of abdomen (Fig. 1) shows absence of left kidney in left renal fossa. The left renal fossa shows bowel loops. Right kidney appears normal. No ectopic kidney was seen. Findings suggest left renal aplasia.

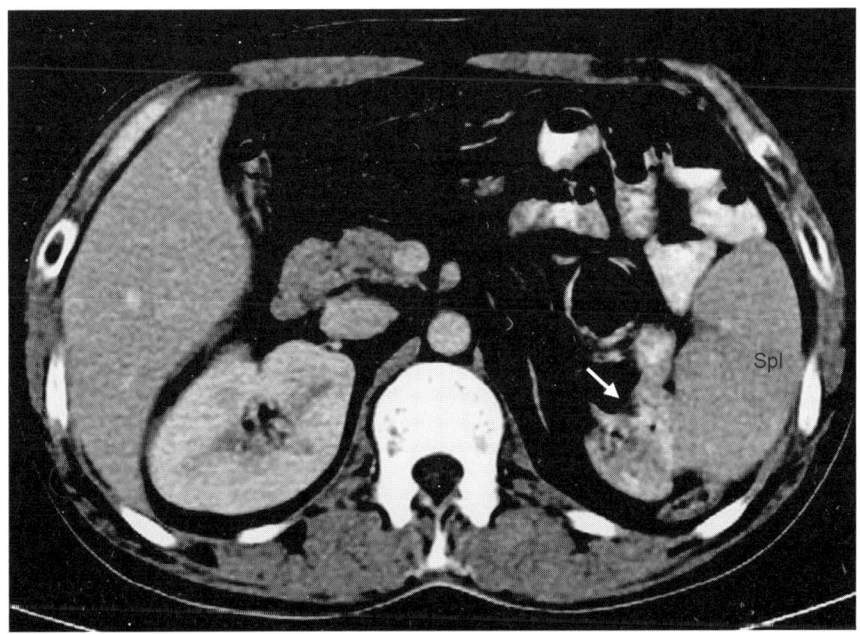

Fig. 1

Comments and Explanation

Renal agenesis refers to a congenital absence of one or both kidneys. If bilateral, the condition is fatal, whereas if unilateral, patients can have a normal life expectancy. If one kidney is absent the other kidney is hypertrophied since it takes over the function. Patients are asymptomatic and diagnosed only when they are screened for some other purpose.

Opinion

Unilateral renal agenesis.

Clinical Discussion

Embryologically renal agenesis results from a failure of the proper development of the metanephros (precursor of adult kidney) resulting in complete absence of a renal structure. Abnormalities in the mesonephros may result not only in renal agenesis (due to absence of induction of the metanephros by the ureteral bud) but also internal genital malformations [due to failure of the Wolffian and Müllerian duct to develop or to involute (according to sex)]. There have been reports of ipsilateral genital abnormalities in 20–70% of cases of renal agenesis. While the incidence of unilateral renal agenesis is not known it is likely 4–20 times more common than bilateral renal agenesis. Unilateral renal agenesis may have other associated birth defects like Müllerian duct anomalies, utero-vaginal aplasia and Potter syndrome.

CASE 65

Dysplastic Kidney

CASE

A 7-year-old female child with pain in left lumbar region was referred to radiology department for CT abdomen.

Radiological Findings on CT Examination

Contrast enhanced CT (Figs 1A to C) shows normal sized right kidney with good excretion of contrast, left kidney is small and dysplastic with multiple well defined cysts of various sizes. There is no evidence of contrast excretion in left kidney. USG shows multiple well defined noncommunicating cysts of various sizes and lack of normal corticomedullary differentiation of left kidney (Fig. 1D).

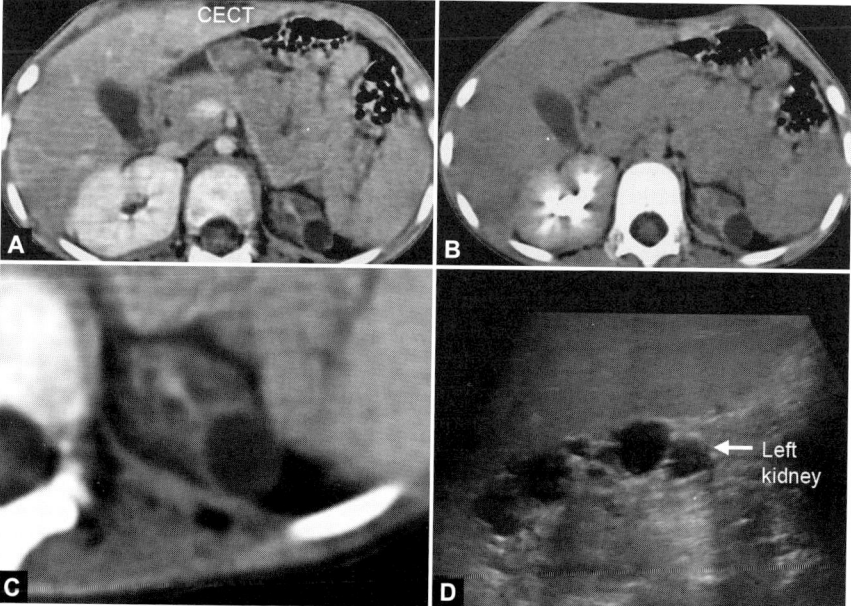

Figs 1A to D

Comments and Explanation

Multicystic dysplastic kidney (MCDK) is a type of pediatric cystic renal disease. It results in multiple small cysts being formed *in utero* in the affected kidney. MCDK develops *in utero* and the diagnosis is often made either antenatally or in the early neonatal period on ultrasound. The vast majority of cases are sporadic and nonfamilial. Rarely autosomal dominant forms are seen. Associated contralateral renal tract abnormalities are common and include vesicoureteric reflux, pelviureteric junction obstruction, horseshoe kidney, ureterocele, and renal hypoplasia. Bilateral MCDK is seen in 19% and contralateral agenesis is seen in 11% patients.

Opinion

Multicystic dysplastic kidney.

Clinical Discussion

The diagnosis of MCDK is often made antenatally with multiple small cysts becoming evident as early as the 15th weeks of gestation. Patient may present with recurrent urinary tract infection, intermittent abdominal pain and sometimes failure to thrive. On USG the kidney shows multiple cysts which are mostly randomly positioned, but may sometimes be peripheral, variable in size and noncommunicating. Sometimes artifacts may make noncommunicating cysts appear to be communicating. The parenchyma is seen in small islands between the cysts and the outline of the kidney tends to be lost. The central sinus complex is absent. Particularly useful, the hydronephrotic form to assess for associated obstructive uropathy. DTPA scan may show some flow to the kidney and possible cortical uptake, but no excretion. The MCDK can be distinguished from hydronephrosis by observing that the fluid filled cysts do not communicate, whereas in hydronephrosis the fluid filled, dilated calyces can be seen to communicate with the renal pelvis and infundibula. Voiding cystourethrogram should be performed to rule out vesicoureteral reflux on the contralateral side, to prevent progressive damage to the functioning kidney. Currently most cases of unilateral MCDK are managed non surgically and are followed with serial USG. The affected kidney may remain unchanged but it frequently undergoes spontaneous regression.

CASE 66

Polycystic Kidneys

CASE

A 40-year-old male presented to the department of radiology with pain in abdomen and raised serum creatinine level, was subjected to CT abdomen.

Radiological Findings on CT Scan

Coronal post contrast reconstructed CT image (Fig. 1) show multiple well defined cysts of varying sizes in both kidneys. The normal renal parenchyma interspaced between the cysts and shows adequate contrast enhancement. Multiple cysts are also seen in liver. These findings are suggestive of bilateral polycystic kidneys.

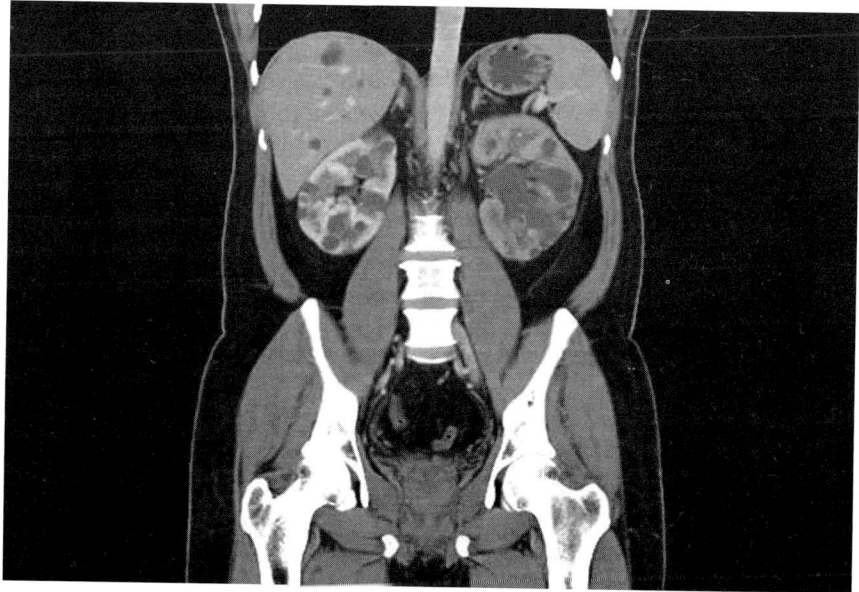

Fig. 1

Comments and Explanation

Adult polycystic kidney disease, which affects approximately 1 in 1000 people, is transmitted as an autosomal dominant trait. Cysts arise from the nephrons and collecting tubules; microdissection reveals that the cysts communicate directly with the nephrons and collecting tubules. Islands of normal parenchymal renal tissue are interspaced between the cysts. Ultrasound is an excellent choice for repeated imaging as it is relatively inexpensive and lacks ionising radiation. Simple renal cysts will appear rounded, anechoic with well-defined imperceptible walls and posterior acoustic enhancement with very thin regular and imperceptible, wall. CT is sensitive to characterize the diagnosis of renal cysts. Simple cysts appear as structures with near water attenuation.

Cysts which have had internal complications may be hyperattenuating, with internal nonenhancing septations or calcifications. A complex cystic mass with solid components or thick septa which enhance should be viewed with suspicion, and presence of a renal cell carcinoma suspected. Calcification may develop. Renal cell carcinomas in contrast, although usually cystic in the setting of autosomal dominant polycystic kidney disease (ADPKD), will have solid components of thick septa with blood flow. Autosomal dominant polycystic kidney disease (ADPKD) is an inherited condition that causes small, fluid-filled sacs called cysts to develop in the kidneys. Although children are born with the condition, ADPKD does not usually cause any noticeable problems until the cysts grow large enough to affect the kidneys' functions. In most cases, this does not occur until 30–60 years of age.

Opinion

Polycystic kidney disease.

Clinical Discussion

Clinical presentation is variable and includes dull flank pain, abdominal or flank masses, hematuria and hypertension. A number of conditions are well recognized as being associated with ADPKD like cerebral Berry's aneurysm, intracranial dolichoectasia, aortic dissection and colonic diverticulosis. The kidneys are normal at birth, and with time develop multiple cysts. At the age of 30 years, approximately 68% of patients will have visible cysts by ultrasound. Patients present with hypertension and progressive renal failure after their third decade of life. Autosomal dominant polycystic kidney disease (ADPKD) is uncommon in children and is rarely seen in neonates. Renal complications that can occur are progression to end stage renal failure, recurrent urinary infection, cyst, hemorrhage or infection resulting in acute pain and cyst rupture resulting in retroperitoneal hemorrhage.

CASE 67

Pelviureteric Junction Obstruction

CASE

A 35-year-old male with history of severe right flank pain was referred to department of radiology for CT scan abdomen.

Radiological Findings on CT Examination

Axial and coronal reconstructed post contrast CT images of abdomen (Figs 1A and B) shows calculus in right proximal ureter with gross dilatation of pelvicalyceal

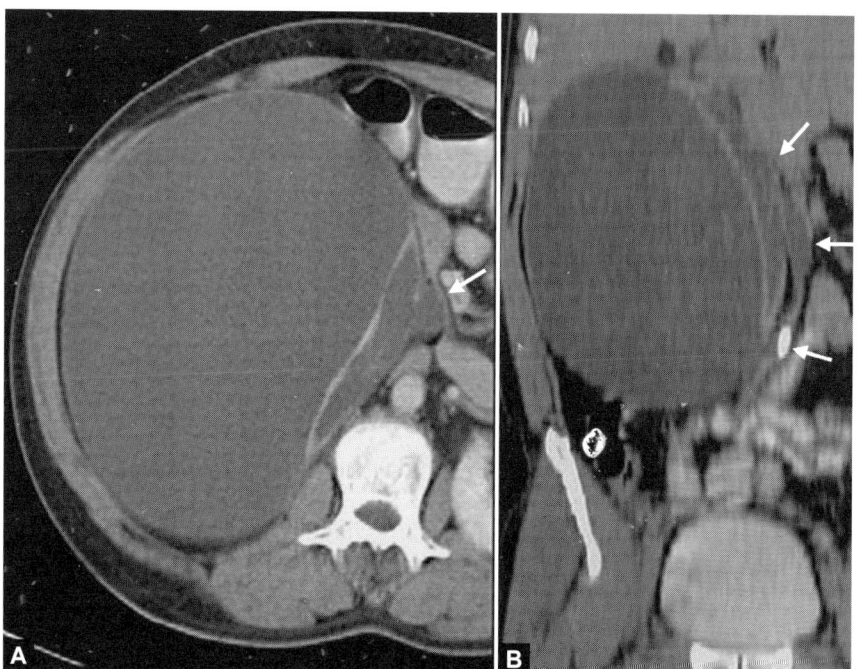

Figs 1A and B

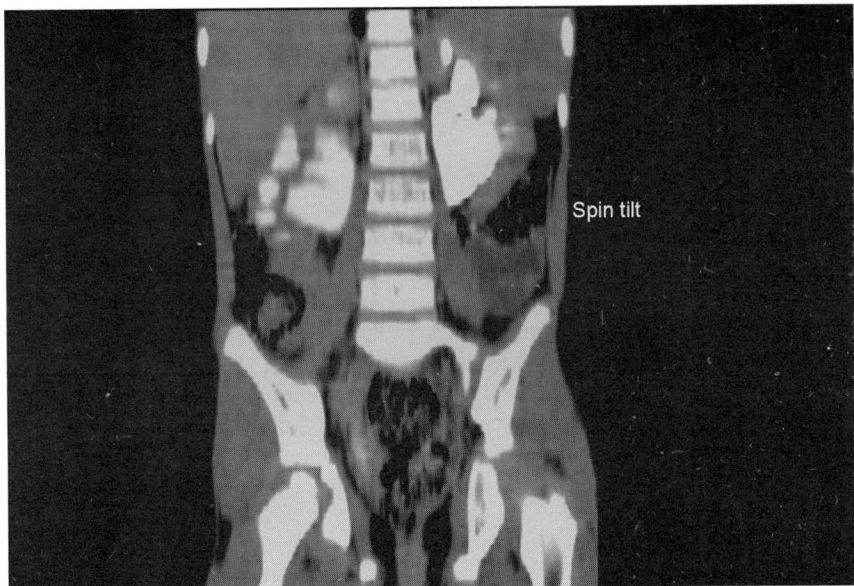

Fig. 2

system and severe thinning of renal parenchyma. Findings suggest obstructive uropathy.

In another patient post contrast CT coronal reconstructed image (Fig. 2) shows bilateral dilatated pelvicalyceal system with abrupt narrowing at pelviureteric junction in a case of bilateral pelviureteric junction obstruction.

Comments and Explanation

Obstruction at the pelviureteric junction (PUJ) leads to proximal hydronephrosis. The amount of obstruction governs the changes in renal pelvicalyceal system. In complete obstruction there will be severe dilatation of pelvicalyceal system with loss of renal parenchyma. Renal calculi is one of the most common causes of pelviureteric junction obstruction. If the calculus remains impacted at that site for a longer period leads to obstructive uropathy. Routinely intravenous urogram (IVU) has been performed for assessing for PUJ obstruction. Ultrasound will often show a dilated renal pelvis with a collapsed proximal ureter. CT may show evidence of hydronephrosis with collapsed ureters and is useful for assessing crossing vessels at the PUJ especially when surgical intervention is planned. Scintigraphy can quantitate the degree of obstruction.^{99m}Tc MAG3 is the agent of choice. Diuretic (Furosemide) renogram is performed to evaluate between obstructive vs nonobstructive hydronephrosis. PUJ "obstruction" will demonstrate excretion (downward slope on renogram) after administration of diuretic from the collecting system. Whereas mechanical obstructive hydronephrosis will demonstrate no downward slope on renogram, with retained tracer in collecting system.

Opinion

Pelviureteric junction obstruction with calculus.

Clinical Discussion

Pelviureteric junction (PUJ) obstruction is defined as an obstruction of the flow of urine from the renal pelvis to the proximal ureter. The resultant back pressure within the renal pelvis may lead to progressive renal damage and deterioration. Congenital causes include abnormal muscle arrangement at PUJ, ischemic insult to PUJ region, urothelial ureteric fold. Causes in adults include preceeding renal pelvic trauma, obstructing calculus distal to PUJ, previous pyelitis with scarring, intrinsic malignancy, extrinsic ureter compression of encasement, fibrosis, malignancy. Patient is usually known case of renal calculus, in which the calculus gets dislodged from kidney and gets stuck at the PUJ. Patient presents with severe flank pain, hematuria. Pain radiates towards the thighs, scrotum or sometimes to back. The pain increases on excess fluid intake due to fullness of pelvicalyceal system. In these cases early diagnosis is necessary since once renal damage is done, then removing the calculus won't help kidney to gain function. Dynamic contrast-enhanced magnetic resonance urography (MRU) is the latest imaging modality used in assessing PUJ obstruction. In children, this study offers the advantages of no radiation exposure and excellent anatomical and functional details with a single study. The study also provides details of renal vasculature, renal pelvis anatomy, location of crossing vessels, renal cortical scarring, and ureteral fetal folds in the proximal ureter.

CASE 68
Obstructive Uropathy

CASE 1 RENAL PELVIC CALCULUS

A 35-year-old female presented to the department of radiology with pain in left flank region and hematuria.

Radiological Findings on CT Examination

Plain radiograph (Fig. 1A) shows a calculus in left paravertebral region at the level of L1-L2 intervertebral disc space.

Plain and post contrast axial CT image (Figs B and C) confirms the position of calculus. The calculus is seen in left renal pelvis with dilatation of pelvicalyceal system. Excretory phase shows contrast in dilated renal pelvis and calyces. Contrast density obscures the calculus (Fig. 1D).

Comments and Explanation

Renal pelvic calculus is due to minerals crystallizing out of urine in a normal urinary tract. Over 90% of calculi are radiopaque on plain films and virtually all are picked up on CT. They contain calcium salts, usually a mixture of oxalate and phosphate, sometimes pure phosphate or oxalate. The hallmark of obstruction on USG is the presence of hydronephrosis. Prominent anechoic structures within the renal sinus represent a dilated pelvicalyceal system. Renal calculi may be demonstrated as echogenic foci with or without shadowing, small ureteral stones are extremely difficult to detect. Unenhanced helical CT has both a high sensitivity and a high specificity in detecting ureteral calculi in the acute setting. Dilatation of the pelvicalyceal system is seen on CT as anterior and medial bulging of the renal pelvis, which is of low attenuation compared to the surrounding renal parenchyma. Renal enlargement also may be observed in some patients. Perinephric fat stranding, representing engorged lymphatics and/or edema, is seen as linear wispy densities in the normally low-attenuation fat. Moderate-to-severe perinephric stranding generally corresponds to the degree of obstruction present.

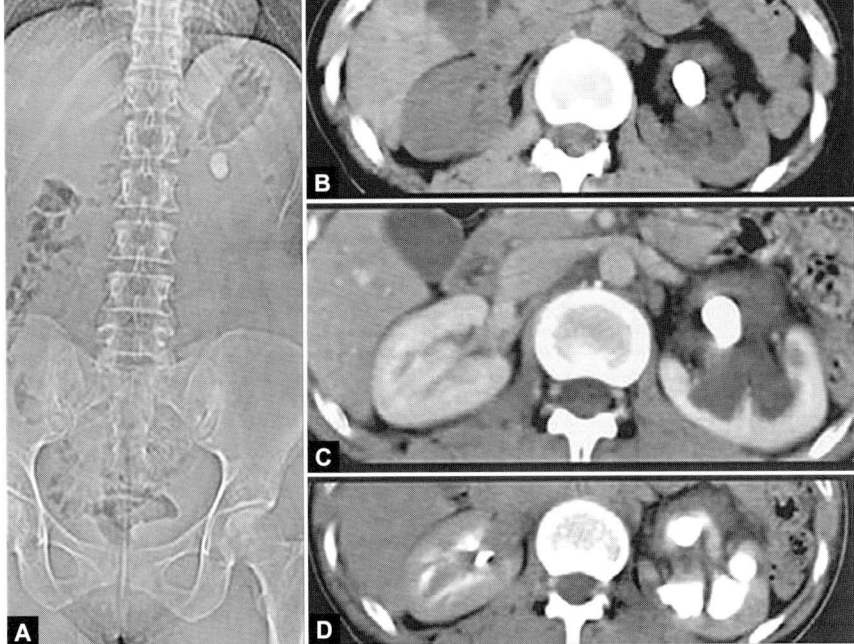

Figs 1A to D

Opinion

Left renal pelvic calculus.

Clinical Discussion

Acute onset of severe flank pain radiating to the groin, gross or microscopic hematuria, nausea, and vomiting not associated with an acute abdomen are symptoms that most likely indicate renal colic caused by an acute ureteral or renal pelvic obstruction from a calculus. Location and quality of pain are related to position of the stone within the urinary tract. Severity of pain is related to the degree of obstruction, presence of ureteral spasm, and presence of any associated infection.

Renal colic has been described as having 3 clinical phases. The first phase is the acute or onset phase. The second phase is the constant phase. The third phase is the abatement or relief phase.

Treatment for acute episode is with non-steroidal anti-inflammatory drugs (NSAIDs). Definitive treatment is in the form of surgical removal of calculus or extracorporeal shock wave lithotripsy (ESWL).

CASE 2 STAGHORN CALCULI

A 33-year-old male came to the radiology department with complaints of pain in bilateral lumbar regions since 2 months.

Radiological Findings on CT Examination

Plain CT axial sections show bilateral renal calculi in the pelvicalyceal system taking the shape of the pelvicalyceal system suggestive of staghorn calculi. There is bilateral hydronephrosis with thinning of renal cortex. Small nonobstructive left renal calyceal calculus is also seen (Figs 2A and B).

Comments and Explanation

Staghorn calculi are the result of recurrent infection and are thus more commonly encountered in women, those with renal tract anomalies, spinal cord injuries, neurogenic bladder or ileal ureteral diversion. The majority of staghorn calculi are symptomatic, presenting with fever, hematuria, flank pain and potentially septicemia and abscess formation. On X-ray the vast majority of staghorn calculi are radiopaque and appear as branching calcific densities overlying the renal outline and may mimic an excretory phase IVP. Lamination within the stone is common. The collecting system is filled with a densely calcific mass producing intense posterior acoustic shadowing on ultrasound. On CT, staghorn calculi are radiopaque and conform to the renal pelvis and calyces, which are often to some degree dilated. When viewed on bone windows they have a laminated appearance, due to alternating bands of magnesium ammonium phosphate and calcium phosphate.

Opinion

Bilateral staghorn calculi.

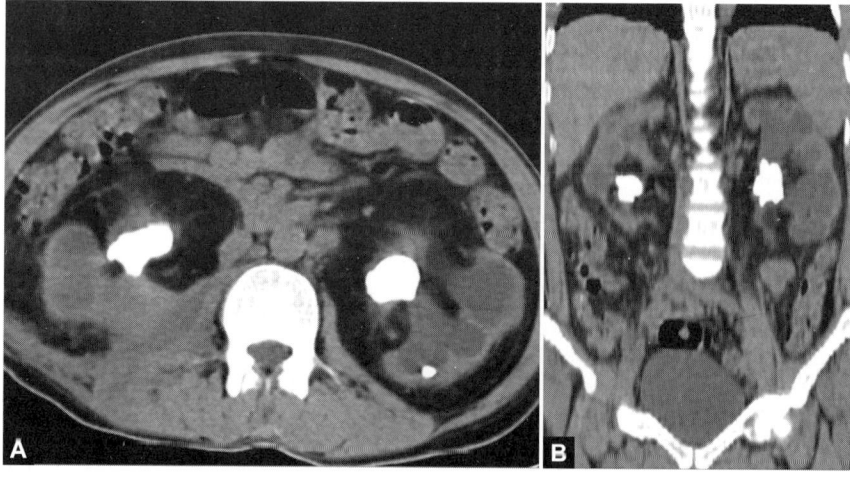

Figs 2A and B

Clinical Discussion

Staghorn calculi represent a less-common nephrolithiasis subgroup so named because the significant stone burden that fills the renal pelvis and calyces forms a shape on radiographs that resembles a deer's horns. Most staghorn stones in Western society are composed of struvite and can cause significant morbidity and mortality if left untreated; therefore, large struvite stones must typically be removed. Unlike other urinary stones that commonly produce symptoms (e.g. renal colic) that necessitate intervention, treatment of **struvite stones often occurs in patients without classic signs of nephrolithiasis; this is because large staghorn calculi may not cause acute renal or ureteral dilatation and resultant pain.

Staghorn calculi need to be treated surgically (PCNL +/- ESWL) and the entire stone removed, including small fragments, as otherwise these residual fragments act as a reservoir for infection and recurrent stone formation. If left untreated, staghorn calculi result in chronic infection and eventually may progress to xanthogranulomatous pyelonephritis.

**Struvite is a phosphate mineral having the formula $NH_4MgPO_4 \cdot 6H_2O$. Struvite calculus form in association with infection. In this *urease* enzyme is produced by some bacteria in the urinary tract which helps with ammonium needed for this type of stone production. These stones have speedy growth resulting in staghorn calculus.

CASE 3 URETERIC CALCULUS

A 40-year-old female patient came with the complaints of pain in both the lumbar region radiating to groin accompanied with hematuria.

Radiological Findings on CT Examination

Plain CT KUB shows a hyperdense focus in the left lower ureter (Fig. 3A) suggestive of lower ureteric calculus with dilatation of the pelvicalyceal system and enlargement of the kidney.

In another patient plain CT scan abdomen (Figs 3B and C) show bilateral hyperdense foci at the vesicoureteric junction with hydronephrosis suggestive of bilateral vesicoureteric junction calculi.

Comments and Explanation

X-ray kidney, ureters, and bladder (KUB) is not very sensitive in detecting calculi as compared to USG and CT. Calculi may be present in 30% of the time when X-ray KUB is negative. Ureteric calculi can be confused with phleboliths on plain X-ray. Typically, phleboliths are round or oval, and they may demonstrate a central lucency. However, they are often difficult to distinguish from ureteric calculi. Phleboliths in the pelvis are usually located lower than and lateral to the ureter. Ultrasound was the previous standard study for ureterolithiasis and is still the best investigation if non-contrast computerized tomography (NCCT) is not available. It provides information regarding site and degree of obstruction and size of stone. Lately it has been replaced by CT. Pelvicaliectasis is noted proximal

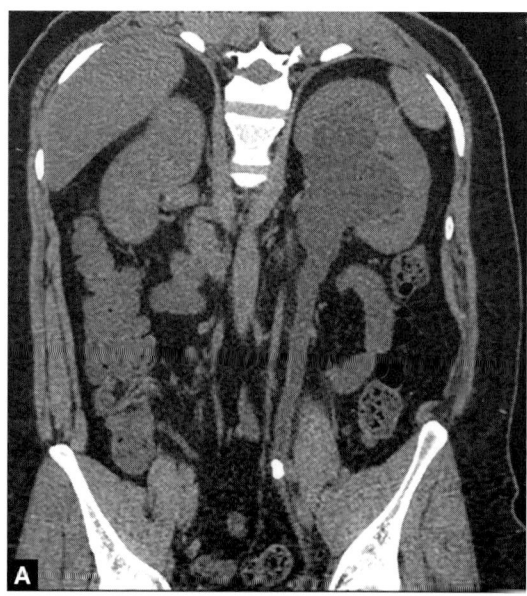

Fig. 3A

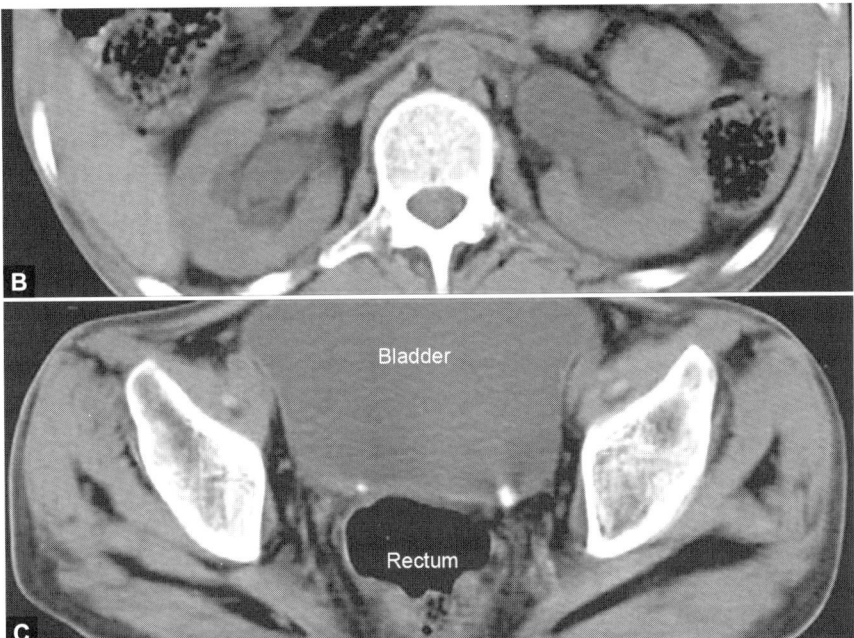

Figs 3B and C

to the obstruction caused by the ureteric calculi. The twinkling artifact sign is seen when color flow is put on the calculus. Absent ureteral jet on affected side may be present with partially obstructing calculus. CT is a highly sensitive, specific and accurate modality for detecting ureteric and vesicoureteric junction calculi. Spiral CT is increasingly replacing IVU in the investigation of ureteric colic and can be regarded as the investigation of choice. It is performed without injection of contrast medium and provides rapid result. The study of choice is nonenhanced abdominal and pelvic CT. In the presence of ureteral calculi, proximal ureterectasis is the most commonly seen indirect sign. The other differential for calculus within the ureter includes phlebolith. The presence of the comet tail sign an adjacent eccentric, tapering soft tissue mass corresponding to the noncalcified portion of a pelvic vein helps differentiate between ureteric calculus and phlebolith. The other indirect signs of vesicoureteric junction calculi on CT are ureterovesical junction edema, stranding of perinephric and paraureteric fat.

Opinion

Bilateral vesicoureteric junction calculi.

Clinical Discussion

Renal colic is characterized by acute colicky flank pain frequently radiating into pelvis, groin and testis and hematuria. Ureteric calculi occur in 12% of the general population. It is much more common in males with a male to female incidence of 4:1. The peak onset occurs in the 3rd decade. The various types of stones include calcium oxalate, struvite, uric acid, calcium phosphate and cystine. Various metabolic conditions that predispose to urinary stones are hypercalciuria, hypoxaluria, hyperuricosuria, cystinuria, xanthinuria and nephrocalcinosis. Most vessels are impacted at narrowest portions of the ureters which are ureteropelvic junction, iliac vessel crossing and vesicoureteric junction. The gold standard imaging investigation is now CT-KUB with a sensitivity rate of 99% for stones as small as 1 mm. Ultrasound is largely reserved for complications such as pyonephrosis and hydronephrosis, which may require percutaneous nephrostomy insertion.

CASE 69

Emphysematous Pyelonephritis

CASE

A 50-year-old diabetic male presented to the department of radiology with flank pain, fever since 4–5 days.

Radiological Findings on CT Examination

Axial post contrast CT image of the abdomen at the level of kidneys shows enlarged left kidney. Multiple nonenhancing areas with air pockets are seen within the left renal parenchyma (Fig. 1). Findings are suggestive of emphysematous pyelonephritis.

Comments and Explanation

Emphysematous pyelonephritis (EPN) is a life-threatening, fulminant, necrotizing upper urinary tract infection associated with gas within the kidney. It is rare, but the frequency is higher in patients who are immunocompromised, especially patients with diabetes. *Escherichia coli* and *Klebsiella pneumoniae* are the most common organisms isolated from urine culture. The diagnosis of emphysematous pyelonephritis (EPN) is established radiologically. Without early therapeutic intervention, the condition becomes rapidly progressive, generalizes to fulminant sepsis, and carries a high mortality rate. CT is the modality of choice for evaluating patients with emphysematous pyelonephritis. Findings include parenchymal enlargement and destruction, small bubbly or linear streaks of gas, fluid collections, gas-fluid levels, and focal tissue necrosis with or without abscess.

Opinion

Emphysematous pyelonephritis.

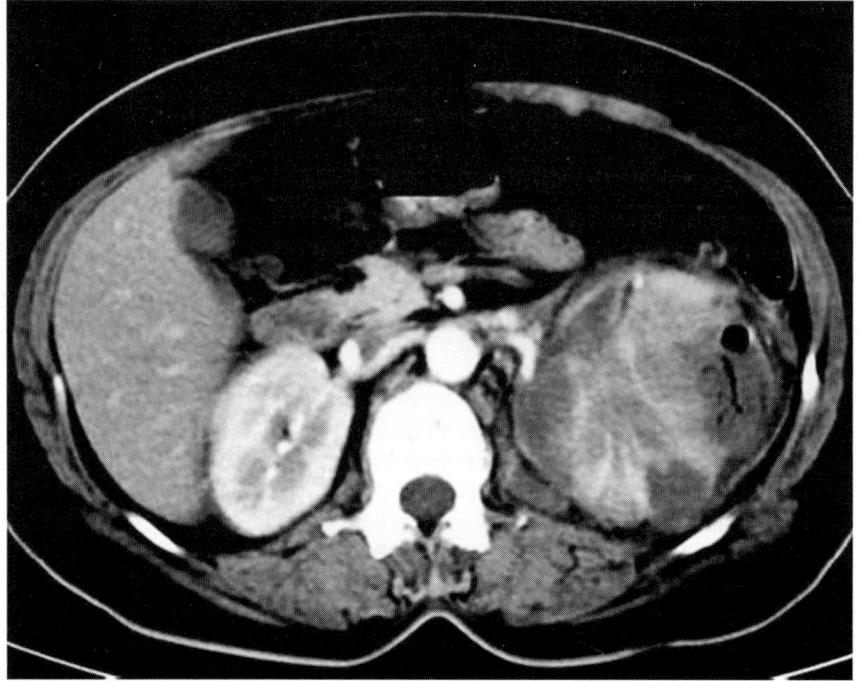

Fig. 1

Clinical Discussion

The mean age of patients with EPN is reported as 55 years, with a range of 19–81 years. The condition is 6 times more common in women. Ninety-five percent of patients have diabetes. In most patients, the diabetes is uncontrolled, with high levels of glycosylated hemoglobin (72%) or high levels of blood sugar. Patients typically present with fever, abdominal or flank pain, nausea and vomiting, dyspnea, acute renal impairment, altered sensorium, shock, and thrombocytopenia. Crepitus over the flank area may occur in advanced cases of EPN. Two types of distribution of the gas have been found to correlate with prognosis. Type 1 emphysematous pyelonephritis is characterized by renal parenchymal destruction that manifests with either streaky or mottled areas of gas. Intra- or extrarenal fluid collections are notably absent. In contradiction, type 2 emphysematous pyelonephritis is characterized by renal or perirenal fluid collections containing loculated gas or gas within the urinary collecting system. Intravenous antibiotics are administered and percutaneous catheter drainage of perirenal or retroperitoneal collections is done. Severe cases often warrant a nephrectomy.

CASE 70

Renal Vein Thrombosis

CASE

A 40-year-old male with acute left flank pain and fever was subjected to CT abdomen.

Radiological Findings on CT Examination

Axial post contrast CT image of abdomen at the level of kidneys shows enlarged left kidney with multiple hypodense nonenhancing areas of collection with multiple air pockets. Left renal vein is stretched and shows an intraluminal filling defect (Fig. 1) suggestive of thrombosis. Findings are suggestive of emphysematous pyelonephritis along with left renal vein thrombosis.

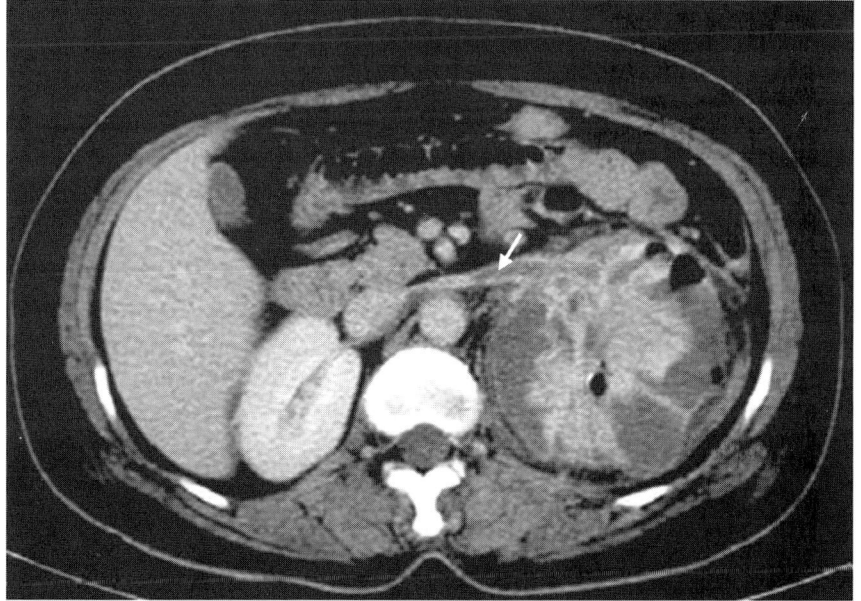

Fig. 1

Comments and Explanation

Renal vein thrombosis (RVT) has numerous etiologies, but most commonly occurs in patients with nephrotic syndrome. Dehydration and sepsis are common underlying factors for renal vein thrombosis in children. In adults, renal vein thrombosis can result from a variety of disorders include renal cell carcinoma, nephrotic syndrome and collagen vascular disease. US is the initial study of choice to exclude the presence of RVT. In an acute setting, US may reveal an edematous and enlarged kidney with decreased echogenicity caused by diffuse edema, as well as focal or diffuse disruption of parenchymal architecture and/or thrombus in the renal vein. CT findings include decreased nephrographic attenuation, loss of corticomedullary differentiation, a low-attenuating thrombus in the renal vein, and renal enlargement with persistent parenchymal opacification. In the acute stage of RVT, capsular venous collaterals and thickening of the Gerota's fascia are often observed. Acute renal vein thrombosis presents as absent nephrogram, enlarged renal outline and stretched pelvicalyceal system.

Opinion

Emphysematous pyelonephritis with partially thrombosed left renal vein.

Clinical Discussion

The presentation of RVT is variable, and patients may be asymptomatic. When RVT occurs as a result of malignancy, the signs of the renal malignancy like hematuria and weight loss predominate. The more common chronic form of RVT is generally overt. The less frequent acute form usually occurs in younger patients, with flank pain and macroscopic hematuria, which can be severe in the acute onset of thrombosis. When RVT is associated with infection then patients present with pain, pyuria, and fever. RVT is seen in associated with antithrombin III deficiency, protein C or S deficiency, antiphospholipid antibody syndrome, pregnancy or estrogen therapy, renal vein invasion by malignant cells, postrenal transplantation, Behçet syndrome, and extrinsic compression. CT currently is the procedure of choice for diagnosing RVT. It depicts the occluded veins and renal changes. Treatment of underlying cause is essential in treating the thrombosis along with anticoagulation therapy. Surgery is rarely needed for treatment.

CASE
71
Renal Laceration

CASE

A 40-year-old male presented to the department of radiology with history of blunt abdominal trauma.

Radiological Findings on CT Examination

Coronal post contrast reconstructed CT image of abdomen at the level of kidneys show a large area of hypodensity in right kidney extending from its lateral border to medial border horizontally. There is evidence of extravasation of contrast from the middle and lower calyceal system. The interpolar region and lower pole of right kidney appear hypodense suggesting large hematoma which is seen to spread into the perirenal spaces (Fig. 1). This is suggestive of large renal tear and Grade 4 renal injury according to American Association for the Surgery of Trauma (AAST).

Comments and Explanation

Renal trauma can result from direct blunt, penetrating and iatrogenic injury. The mechanism of renal trauma is from deceleration injuries from collision of the kidney with the vertebral column or thoracic cage. Renal laceration is seen as irregular linear hypodense parenchymal areas. Most of these lacerations heal on conservative management. Laceration with vascular injury or fracture kidney requires operative intervention.

Opinion

Small renal laceration.

Clinical Discussion

Patients tend to present with microscopic or macroscopic hematuria and flank and/or abdominal pain. In more severe cases, hypotension and shock may be

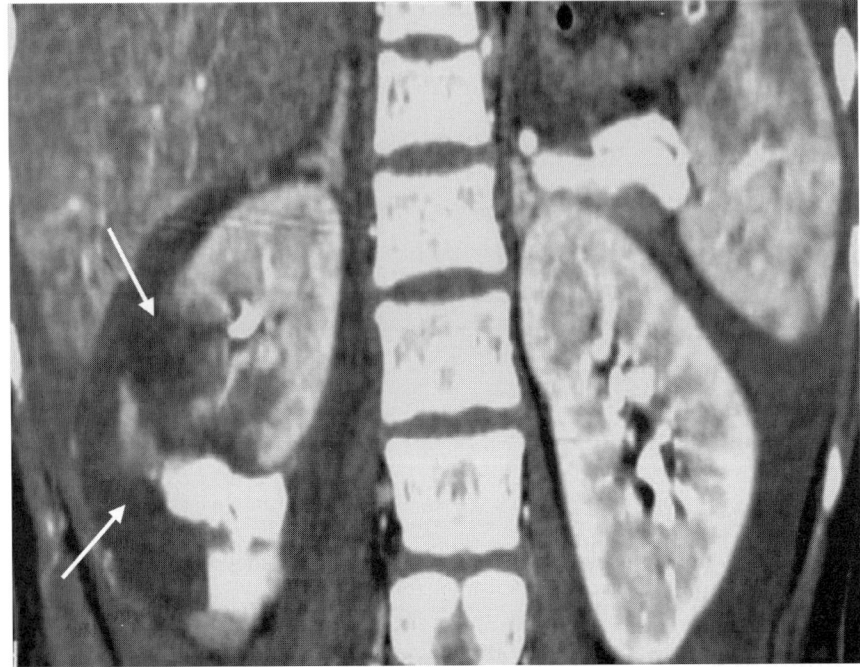

Fig. 1

present. Iatrogenic injuries can result from surgery, percutaneous renal biopsy, nephrostomy and extracorporeal shock wave lithotripsy (ESWL). The mechanism of injury is direct blow (>80%) frequently compressed and often lacerated by lower ribs, and acceleration-deceleration injuries can produce renal artery tears. It is associated with other organ injury in 20% of cases.

Renal injuries are graded by the American Association for the Surgery of Trauma (AAST) on the basis of the depth of injury and the involvement of vessels or the collecting system as follows:
- *Grade 1:* Hematuria with normal imaging studies, contusions, nonexpanding subcapsular hematomas.
- *Grade 2:* Nonexpanding perinephric hematomas confined to the retroperitoneum, superficial cortical lacerations less than 1 cm in depth without collecting system injury.
- *Grade 3:* Renal lacerations greater than 1 cm in depth that do not involve the collecting system.
- *Grade 4:* Renal lacerations extending through the kidney into the collecting system, injuries involving the main renal artery or vein with contained hemorrhage, segmental infarctions without associated lacerations, expanding subcapsular hematomas compressing the kidney.
- *Grade 5:* Shattered or devascularized kidney, ureteropelvic avulsions, complete laceration or thrombus of the main renal artery or vein.

CASE 72

Renal Angiomyolipoma

CASE

A 29-year-old female patient came with history of pain in abdomen and was referred to radiology department for CT scan.

Radiological Findings on CT Examination

CT scan (Figs 1A to C) shows multiple well defined lesions containing fat, internal septae and soft tissue components in both kidneys. The soft tissue components show mild enhancement. The lesion at upper pole of left kidney has displaced the pancreas and splenic vein anteriorly.

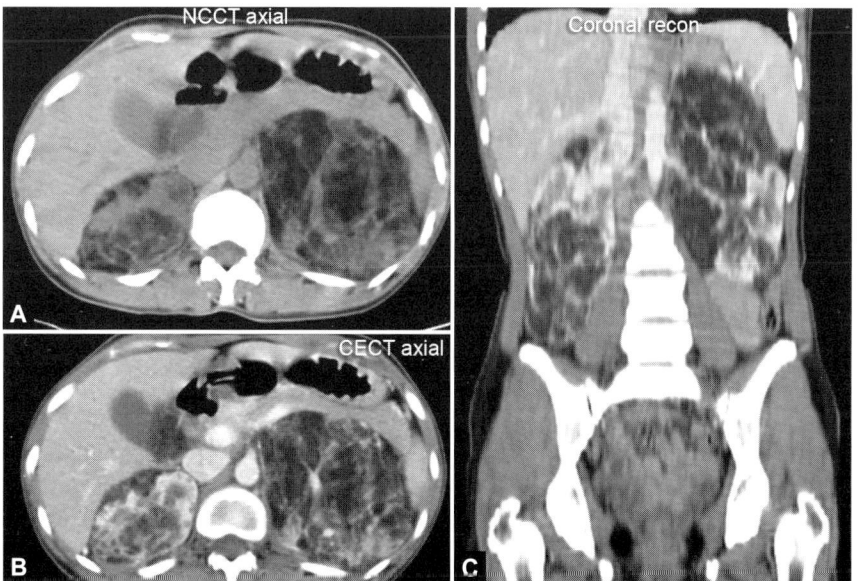

Figs 1A to C

Comments and Explanation

Renal angiomyolipomas (AML) are benign renal neoplasms. They are composed of blood vessels (angio), plump spindle cells (myo) and adipose tissue (lipo). On USG angiomyolipomas appear as well defined hyperechoic lesions, located in the cortex with posterior acoustic shadowing. In the setting of tuberous sclerosis, they may be so numerous that the entire kidney is affected, appearing echogenic with loss of normal corticomedullary differentiation. On CT it appears as well-marginated, cortical-based, heterogeneous tumor predominantly of fat density (-20 to -40 HU) and shows variable enhancement due to smooth muscle and vessels. Angiomyolipomas >4 cm bleed spontaneously in 60% cases. In the setting of hemorrhage, or when lesions contain little fat, appearances may be difficult to distinguish from a renal cell carcinoma. Isolated reports of renal cell carcinoma with demonstrable fat content have appeared in the literature. These renal carcinomas may entrap surrounding perinephric fat or undergo fatty change because of metaplasia. Intratumoral fat is also reported in Wilms tumors, oncocytoma, xanthogranulomatous pyelonephritis, renal and retroperitoneal liposarcoma, and teratoma. Hemorrhagic shock can occur from bleeding into angiomyolipoma or into retroperitoneum.

Opinion

Bilateral renal angiomyolipomas.

Clinical Discussion

The majority of angiomyolipomas are typically seen in adults in fifth decade of life with a strong female predilection. Angiomyolipomas occur in 80% of patients with tuberous sclerosis and are large, bilateral and usually multiple. Small lesions are asymptomatic. Acute abdominal pain due to hemorrhage is the most common presenting symptom. Patient may have a palpable mass with hematuria. Although many angiomyolipomas do not show growth over time, those that occur with the tuberous sclerosis complex are more likely to show progressive evolution and are more likely to need intervention such as selective arterial embolization, renal sparing surgery, or nephrectomy. The need for intervention, including prophylactic embolization, should be predicated on the presence of rapid growth or the development of symptoms related to retroperitoneal hemorrhage and mass effect. Annual follow-up is required for lesions <4 cm. Larger tumors or those that have been symptomatic can be electively embolized or resected with a partial nephrectomy.

CASE 73

Wilms' Tumor

CASE

A 6-year-old male child presented to the department of radiology with gradually increasing lump in abdomen.

Radiological Findings on CT Examination

Axial post contrast CT images of abdomen (Figs 1A to D) at the level of kidneys show a large well-defined enhancing soft tissue density lesion with few areas of

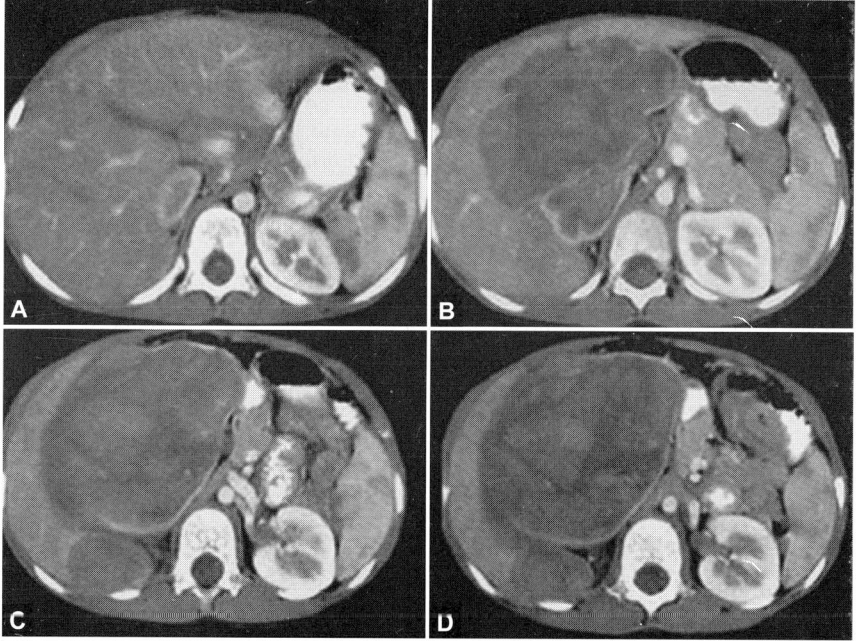

Figs 1A to D

necrosis, involving the right kidney, sparing its upper pole. Medially, the lesion is seen to displace the pancreas and great vessels to left side with compression of IVC. Cranially, the lesion is seen insinuating the inferior surface of liver and inferiorly extends up to iliac crest. Findings are suggestive of Wilms' Tumor.

Comments and Explanation

Wilms' tumor (nephroblastoma) accounts for 87% of pediatric renal masses and arises from mesodermal precursors of the renal parenchyma (metanephros) and occasionally is found to arise in the extrarenal retroperitoneum, presumably within mesonephric remnants. Wilms' tumor is the most common solid renal mass and abdominal malignancy of childhood, with a prevalence of 1 case per 10,000 population. At USG, the mass has heterogeneous echogenicity, which represents hemorrhage, fat, necrosis, or calcification. Examination of the inferior vena cava is critical to detect tumor extension, which could necessitate modification of the surgical approach. CT demonstrates the heterogeneous mass and nodal metastases, as well as areas of calcification and fat. Intravenous administration of contrast material is mandatory to detect nodal or hepatic metastases, tumor extension into the renal vein or inferior vena cava, contralateral synchronous tumor, and associated nephrogenic rests. Wilms' tumor manifests as a solid intrarenal mass with a pseudocapsule and distortion of the renal parenchyma and collecting system. The tumor typically spreads by direct extension and displaces adjacent structures but does not typically encase or elevate the aorta; such encasement or elevation is a distinguishing characteristic of neuroblastoma.

Opinion

Wilms' tumor.

Clinical Discussion

Wilms' tumor is the most common abdominal malignancy of childhood. Both the kidneys are affected synchronously or metachronously. Peak age of incidence is 2.5-3 years. There is no recognized gender predilection; however presentation is a little later in females. Clinical presentation is typically with an asymptomatic painless upper quadrant abdominal mass. Hematuria is seen in approximately 20% of cases and pain is uncommon. It has associations with multiple syndromes. Wilms' tumor staging is largely anatomical and relates to the invasion and spread of the tumor.

The (post-surgical) staging of Wilms' tumor according to the North American National Wilms' Tumor Study Group is summarized below:
- Stage I
  - Confined to kidney
  - Complete resection possible
- Stage II
  - Local spread beyond kidney including renal vein involvement
  - Complete resection possible

- Stage III
  - Lymph-node involvement or
  - *Disease confined to the abdomen:* For example, peritoneal spread, residual tumor
  - Complete resection NOT possible
- Stage IV
  - Hematogenous metastases (typically lungs, liver, distant nodes)
- Stage V
  - Bilateral renal involvement
  - Each kidney should be staged individually

Unilateral Wilms' tumor is generally treated with nephrectomy followed by adjuvant chemotherapy. Presurgical treatment with chemotherapy may be used to promote shrinkage of the tumor and improve outcome. In children with bilateral Wilms' tumor, preoperative chemotherapy is especially important because each kidney is staged separately, and complete resolution of disease in one kidney may allow surgery on the contralateral kidney with eventual cure.

CASE 74

Renal Cell Carcinoma

CASE

A 74-year-old male presented to the department of radiology with painless hematuria and abdominal lump. Patient was subjected to CT scan abdomen and pelvis.

Radiological Findings on CT Examination

CT abdomen shows evidence of iso to hypodense lesion one in both kidneys which show heterogeneous enhancement with central hypodense necrotic areas. Findings suggest bilateral renal cell carcinoma. Multiple well defined hypodense lesions of various sizes are seen in liver. These represent metastases (Figs 1A and B).

In another case axial plain and post contrast CT images of abdomen at the level of kidneys show large, heterogeneously enhancing mass lesion in left renal fossa with central hypodense area suggestive of necrosis (Figs 2A and B). Findings suggest left renal cell carcinoma (RCC). Also chest radiograph and axial post-contrast CT image of thorax shows multiple rounded mass lesions in bilateral lungs suggestive of lung metastases (Figs 2C and D).

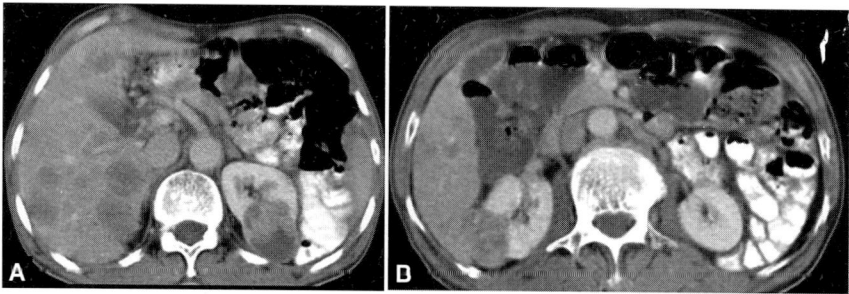

Figs 1A and B

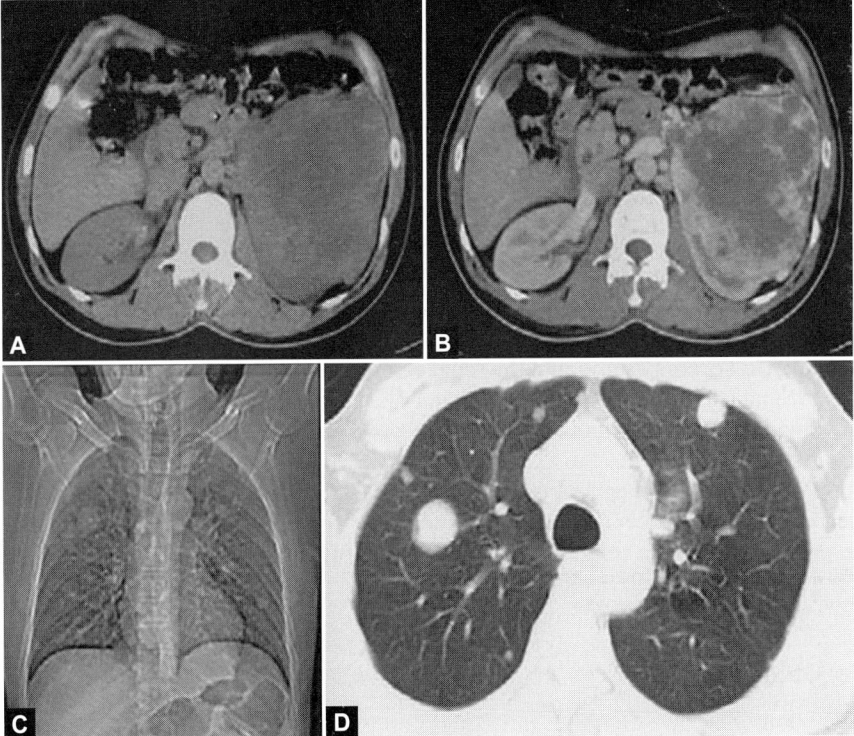

Figs 2A to D

Comments and Explanation

Renal cell carcinoma (RCC) is the most common primary renal malignant neoplasm in adults. It accounts for approximately 90% of renal tumors and 2% of all adult malignancies. Risk factors include increased age, male sex, smoking, cadmium, benzene, trichloroethylene, and asbestos exposure, excessive weight, chronic dialysis use and several genetic syndromes (familial RCC, hereditary papillary RCC, von Hippel-Lindau syndrome, and tuberous sclerosis). It presents as painless hematuria. On CT examination it is iso to hypodense on plain CT and shows heterogeneous enhancement on early arterial phase with necrosis within.

Opinion

Bilateral renal cell carcinoma with metastasis.

Clinical Discussion

Renal cell carcinoma patients are typically 50–70 years of age at presentation, with a moderate male predilection of 2:1. Presentation is classically described as the triad of macroscopic hematuria, flank pain, palpable flank mass. This triad is however only found in 10–15% of patients, and increasingly the diagnosis is being made on CT for assessment of hematuria alone or as an incidental finding. However, clinical symptomatology may be quite nonspecific for example, anorexia, tiredness, weight loss, or fever of unknown origin. Other presentations include varicocele formation from tumor thrombus in the left renal vein or the inferior vena cava. RCC may also present with a variety of paraneoplastic syndromes, such as polycythemia secondary to excessive secretion of erythropoietin, hypercalcemia secondary to factors regulating calcium, and hepatic dysfunction.

RCCs can be staged by using the American Joint Committee on Cancer TNM (T-Tumor, N-Node, M-Metastases) classification, as follows:
- *Stage 1:* RCCs are 7 cm or smaller and confined to the kidney.
- *Stage 2:* RCCs are larger than 7 cm but still organ confined.
- *Stage 3:* Tumors extend into the renal vein or vena cava, involve the ipsilateral adrenal gland and/or perinephric fat, or have spread to local lymph nodes.
- *Stage 4:* Tumors extend beyond the Gerota fascia, have spread to local or distant nodes, or have distant metastases.

Typically in renal cell carcinomas whenever feasible a radical nephrectomy is performed, however in elderly patients or those with comorbidities, and especially those with smaller tumors suggestive of papillary histology, then organ sparing treatment can be done.

SECTION 16

Urinary Bladder

75. Vesical Calculus
76. Urinary Bladder Diverticulum
77. Cystitis
78. Carcinoma Urinary Bladder

CASE 75

Vesical Calculus

CASE

A 40-year-old male with history of burning micturition and pain in the suprapubic region was referred to radiology department for CT abdomen and pelvis.

Radiological Findings on CT Examination

CT pelvis shows calcific lesion (CT value 730 HU) with irregular margins within the urinary bladder diagnosed as vesical calculus (Fig. 1).

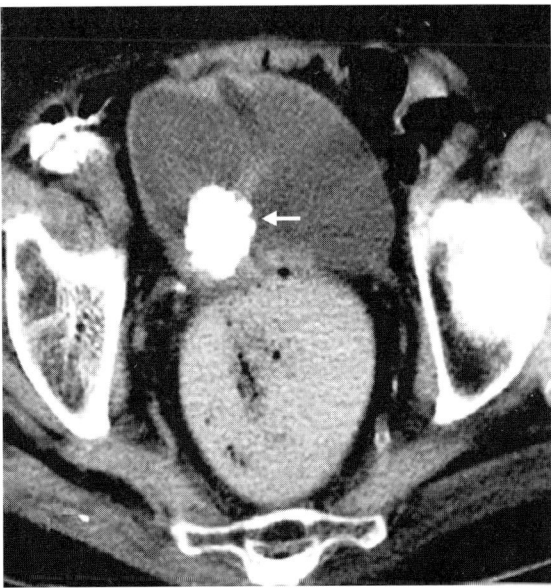

Fig. 1

Comments and Explanation

Initial imaging choice is plain radiography of the kidneys, ureters, and bladder (KUB) area or as the first film of intravenous pyelography (IVP), to detect radiopaque stones. Pure uric acid and ammonium urate stones are radiolucent but may be coated with a layer of opaque calcium sediment. Calculi with laminations are common, with the layers stratified according to metabolic and infectious status. Radiolucent calculi are seen as a filling defect in the bladder on IVP. If the filling defect moves when the patient is repositioned, the presence of a stone is likely possibility. Nonmobile filling defects could be calculi attached to the bladder wall in a diverticulum, differential diagnosis includes urothelial carcinoma, or clot. IVP may also be used to identify associated abnormalities, e.g. upper urinary tract calculi, ureterocele, cystocele, enlarged prostate, and bladder diverticula.

USG is widely available; being rapid modality is extensively used in the diagnosis of bladder calculi. Sonograms typically show a classic hyperechoic object with posterior shadowing, and they are effective in identifying both radiolucent and radiopaque stones.

CT is usually performed for other reasons like abdominal pain, pelvic mass or suspected abscess and may demonstrate bladder calculi even without intravenous contrast. Unenhanced spiral CT scanning is highly sensitive and specific in diagnosing calculi along the urinary tract. Even pure urate calculi can be detected with this method. The stone may be obscured if contrast has been administered.

Opinion

Vesical calculus.

Clinical Discussion

Vesical calculi are common in developing countries. It usually occurs in patients who have urinary stasis, and recurrent bladder infections. It mostly affects males over 50 who have bladder outlet obstruction due to enlarged prostate. The chronic presence of bladder calculi has been associated with squamous cell carcinoma. There may be pain, dysuria, increased frequency, hesitation, terminal gross hematuria, suprapubic fullness. Most bladder stones form from a nidus inside the bladder. They may be single or multiple. Causes include bladder outlet obstruction, urinary infections, neurogenic bladder and schistosomiasis.

CASE 76

Urinary Bladder Diverticulum

CASE

A 50-year-male patient with history of hematuria was referred to department of radiology for CT abdomen and pelvis.

Radiological Findings on CT Examination

Plain X-ray abdomen shows staghorn calculus in right kidney and a large calculus in bladder area (Fig. 1A). CT demonstrates a large posterior bladder diverticulum with a large calculus (Fig. 1B). A large staghorn calculus is seen in right kidney (Fig. 1C). Sagittal reconstructed CT image shows a posterior diverticulum filled with urine and a large calculus within it (Fig. 1D).

Comments and Explanation

A bladder diverticulum is an outpouching from the bladder wall, where mucosa herniates through the bladder wall. They may be solitary or multiple in nature and can vary considerably in size. Diverticula may be congenital or acquired. Acquired diverticula are common, resulting from chronic bladder outlet obstruction. Diverticula are often an incidental finding on imaging investigations, including ultrasound, CT, MRI and IVU. They may be associated with a range of complications including infection, reflux, stone formation and malignancy.

Opinion

Urinary bladder diverticulum with calculus.

Clinical Discussion

A Hutch diverticulum is a congenital bladder diverticulum seen at vesicoureteric junction. Congenital bladder diverticulum, not associated with posterior urethral valve are seen in boys. Patient presents with repeated urinary tract infection,

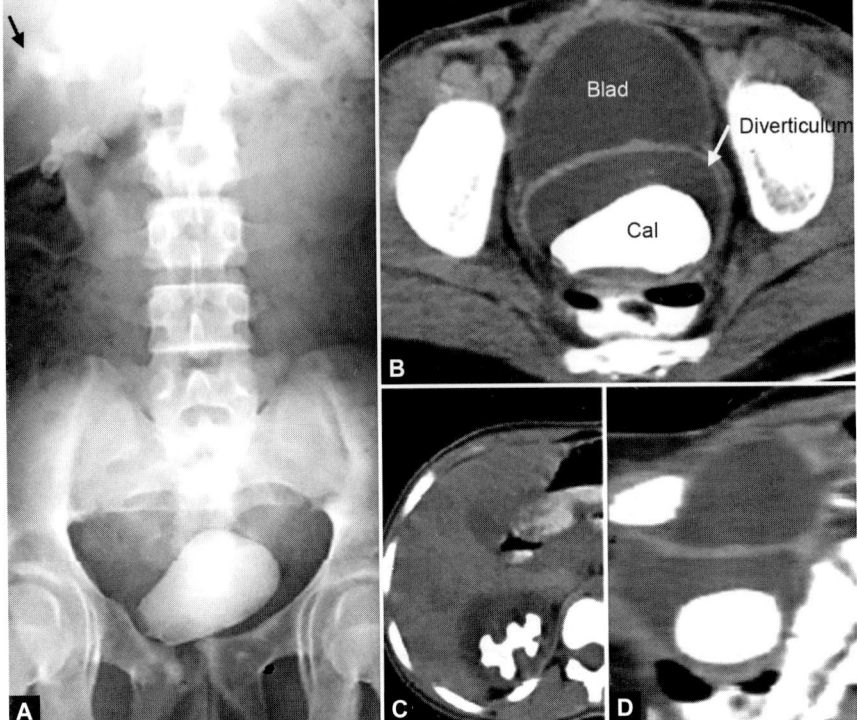

Figs 1A to D

incontinence or urinary retention. Micturating cystourethrogram (MCU) shows contrast filled outpouchings arising from urinary bladder at vesicoureteric junction, and often seen with vesico-ureteric reflux. On USG a round or oval anechoic fluid collection is seen arising from base of urinary bladder or around ureteric orifice. Incidentally detected diverticulum, does not require any therapy. If associated with vesicoureteric reflux, recurrent urinary tract infection (UTI) or obstruction, it should be excised. Differential diagnosis include bladder ears, which protrude through internal inguinal ring. It is more often seen in children than adults. Seen most often when bladder is maximally distended. Bladder ear will empty when bladder is emptied whereas diverticula tend to fill when bladder is emptied.

CASE 77

Cystitis

CASE

A 65-year-old male patient came to the radiology department with history of burning micturition and was subjected to CT scan abdomen.

Radiological Findings on CT Examination

Figure 1 CT scan abdomen and pelvis shows thick irregular enhancing urinary bladder wall s/o cystitis.

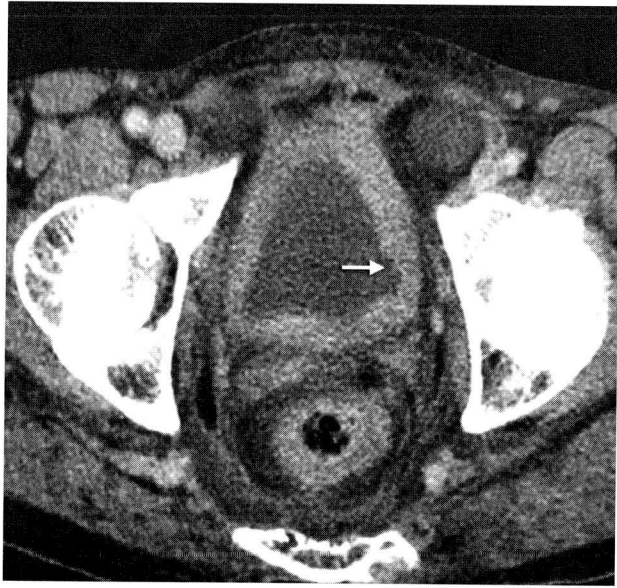

Fig. 1

Comments and Explanation

Cystitis is inflammation of part or the entire urinary bladder wall. It may be described as acute, chronic, hemorrhagic, bullous, emphysematous, polypoid. USG shows thickening of the wall of the bladder when distended (>6 mm). CT shows bladder wall thickening and perivesical edema. MR demonstrates mucosal edema and inflammation as high signal intensity on T2WI, easily differentiated from normal low-signal bladder wall. The common causes are infections, bacterial, viral and fungal. Other causes included are indwelling catheter, calculus, toxic and allergic etiologies.

Opinion

Cystitis.

Clinical Discussion

Acute cystitis may have a normal appearance; chronic usually appears as thickened walls and diminishes filling capacity. Focal inflammation such as bullous edema may be radiographically indistinguishable from bladder carcinoma. Cystitis cystica is characterized by multiple fluid-filled submucosal cysts. Most cases are associated with bladder infection. Cystitis glandularis is a further progression of cystitis cystica with proliferation of mucous secreting glands in the lamina propria. The cysts vary in size and may obstruct the ureteral orifice. Cystitis glandularis may be a precursor of adenocarcinoma of the bladder. Bullous edema of the bladder wall is usually associated with chronic irritation from indwelling catheters. Grape-like cysts elevate the mucosa. Interstitial cystitis is a chronic, idiopathic inflammation of the bladder found most often in women. The bladder capacity is progressively diminished, and the bladder wall thickens and becomes trabeculated and fibrotic. Hemorrhagic cystitis is characterized by hemorrhage into the mucosa and submucosa. It is caused by bacterial or adenovirus infection. Eosinophilic cystitis is an infiltration of the bladder wall by eosinophils. The cause is uncertain. The bladder wall is greatly thickened and frequently nodular. Emphysematous cystitis is a form of bladder inflammation with gas within the bladder wall. It is associated with poorly controlled diabetes mellitus, bladder outlet obstruction, and infection with *Escherichia coli*, which ferment sugar in the urine to release carbon dioxide and hydrogen gasses. Gas within the bladder lumen is seen with emphysematous cystitis, instrumentation, and vesicocolic fistula.

CASE 78

Carcinoma Urinary Bladder

CASE

A 75-year-old female patient came to the radiology department with painless hematuria since 1 month.

Radiological Findings on CT Examination

Figures 1A to F scout image shows staghorn calculus in right renal pelvis. Plain CT shows staghorn calculus with small renal calyceal calculi. A growth is seen within the bladder on right side. Contrast CT shows uptake of contrast by renal

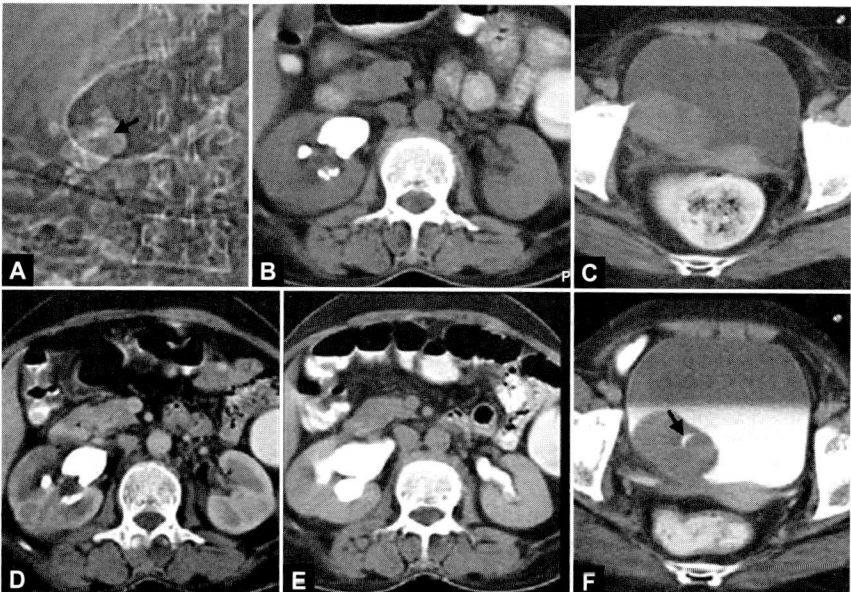

Figs 1A to F

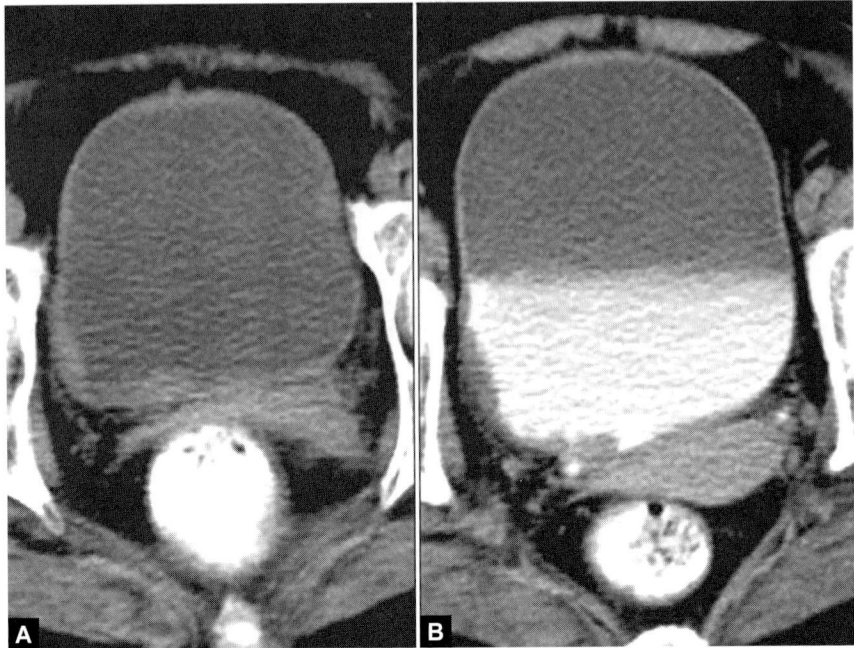

Figs 2A and B

parenchyma and excretion by both kidneys. Delayed contrast CT shows contrast opacified right ureter coursing through the mass in urinary bladder.

In another case (Figs 2A and B) posterior and right lateral wall of urinary bladder shows irregular wall thickening. Right vesicoureteric junction is involved. Fat plane with rectum is however preserved.

Comments and Explanation

Imaging of bladder transitional cell carcinomas has a number of roles: incidental discovery of tumor, tumor staging, tumor staging of locally advanced masses and evaluation of distant metastases and nodal status. Ultrasound has limited role to play in either diagnosis or staging transitional cell carcinomas of the urinary tract in general. On CT bladder transitional cell carcinomas appear as either focal regions of thickening of the bladder wall, or as masses protruding into the bladder lumen, or in advanced cases, extending into adjacent tissues. Care should be taken in assessing bladder wall thickness as these changes with the degree of bladder distension and varies from patient to patient (e.g. patients with bladder outlet obstruction due to benign prostatic hypertrophy). In general however, asymmetric mural thickening should be viewed with suspicion. The masses are of soft tissue attenuation and may be encrusted with small calcifications. Although unable to distinguish between T1, T2 and T3a (microscopic extravesical spread), CT is able to distinguish T3b tumours (stranding/nodules in perivesical fat) and T4 tumours (direct extension into adjacent structures/loss of normal fat plane). Care should be exercised when interpreting stranding or nodularity following transurethral resection or even biopsy, as these changes may be postoperative. Nodal metastases are common. MRI is superior to other modalities in locally staging the tumor. Unfortunately FDG is excreted into the urine, and thus accumulates in the bladder, making it unsuitable for diagnosis of urinary tract tumors.

Opinion

Carcinoma urinary bladder.

Clinical Discussion

The classical clinical presentation is painless gross hematuria. The risk factors being smoking, irradiation, exposure to aniline dyes, chemotherapy with cyclophosphamide. Urothelial (transitional cell carcinomas) are the most common tumors followed by squamous cell carcinomas and adenocarcinomas. Bladder cancer typically occurs in men aged 50–70 years and is related to smoking or occupational exposure to carcinogens. Most urothelial neoplasms are low-grade papillary tumors, which tend to be multifocal and recur but have a relatively good prognosis. High-grade invasive tumors are less common and have a much poorer prognosis. Squamous cell carcinomas and adenocarcinomas occur in the setting of chronic irritation. Rarer mesenchymal tumors include paraganglioma, lymphoma, leiomyoma, and solitary fibrous tumor. A tumor located at the vesicoureteric junction may result in ureteral obstruction and hydronephrosis, which may present with flank pain. Additionally tumors near the urethral orifice may result in bladder outlet obstruction and urinary retention. Occasionally patients only present once systemic symptoms of metastatic disease are present. Diagnosis and local tumor staging is usually achieved with cystoscopy and full thickness biopsy.

SECTION 17

Prostate

79. Carcinoma Prostate

CASE 79

Carcinoma Prostate

CASE

A 60-year-old male patient with prostatomegaly and raised prostate specific antigen (PSA) levels was referred for CT abdomen and pelvis.

Radiological Findings on CT Scan

Prostate is enlarged with irregular contours (Fig. 1A). The fat plane with posterior wall of urinary bladder is lost (Fig. 1B). Enhancing metastases is seen in right lobe of liver (Fig. 1C). Large left pleural effusion with collapse of the underlying lung (Fig. 1D) is seen.

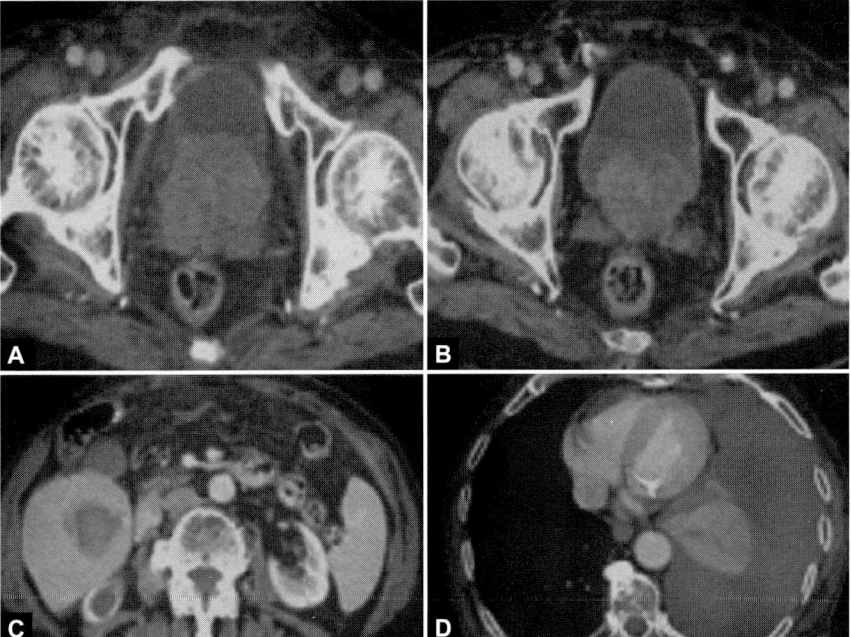

Figs 1A to D

Comments and Explanation

Prostate cancer usually arises within the peripheral zone near the rectum which is why a digital rectal exam (DRE) is a useful screening test. Nowadays serum prostate-specific antigen (PSA) tests and transrectal ultrasound (TRUS)-guided biopsy are widely used for detecting prostate cancers. Few men now present with locoregional or metastatic disease identified by standard imaging, i.e. bone scan or cross-sectional pelvic imaging MRI or CT.

Opinion

Carcinoma prostate with hepatic metastases.

Clinical Discussion

Prostatic carcinoma is the most common malignant tumor in men. Prostatic adenocarcinoma is the most common histological type. Prostate cancer is detected by an elevated prostate specific antigen level (normal range is 1–4 ng/dL). Transrectal ultrasonography (TRUS) is often initially performed in order to detect abnormalities and to guide biopsy, following an abnormal PSA level. On ultrasound prostate cancer is usually seen as a hypoechoic lesion in the peripheral zone of the gland, but can be hyperechoic or isoechoic. USG is used to direct biopsy of suspicious, hypoechoic regions, usually in the peripheral zone. Transrectal ultrasound is also the modality of choice for directing brachytherapy seeds into the prostate gland. USG cannot detect *in situ* prostate cancer. The normal prostate gland appears as an elliptical structure on CT scan. Scans of the abdomen and pelvis are normally obtained prior to the onset of radiation therapy to identify bony landmarks for planning. In advanced disease CT can identify enlarged pelvic and retroperitoneal lymph nodes, hydronephrosis and osteoblastic metastases. The primary indication for MRI of the prostate is in the evaluation of prostate cancer, after an ultrasound guided prostate biopsy has confirmed cancer. MRI using endorectal coil, is considered more sensitive than CT as it can determine extracapsular extension.

SECTION 18

Scrotum

80. Hydrocele
81. Testicular Trauma
82. Seminoma
83. Undescended Testis

CASE 80

Hydrocele

CASE

A 35-year-old male with history of scrotal swelling was referred to the department of radiology for CT abdomen and pelvis.

Radiological Findings on CT Examination

Axial CT pelvis (Fig. 1) shows accumulation of fluid in tunica vaginalis of both testes suggestive of bilateral hydrocele.

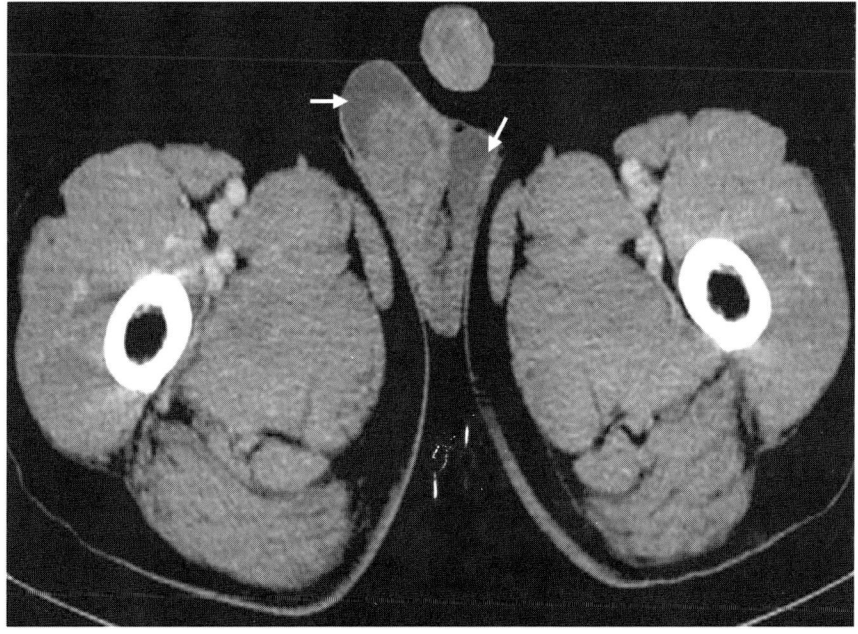

Fig. 1

Comments and Explanation

Ultrasonography provides excellent detail of the testicular parenchyma and is the modality of choice to evaluate hydrocele. It presents as fluid collection surrounding the testis. It may contain septations. Ultrasound is also useful in identifying abnormalities in the testis, complex cystic masses, tumors, appendages, or associated hernia. Plain radiography may be useful for distinguishing an acute hydrocele from an incarcerated hernia. Gas overlying the groin may indicate an incarcerated hernia. On CT examination hydrocele appears as hypodense collection with CT value in HU's similar to water within the scrotal sac. On MRI examination hydrocele is of low intensity on T1WI and high intensity on T2WI.

Opinion

Bilateral hydrocele.

Clinical Discussion

Most hydrocele is acquired and the usual presentation is painless enlarged scrotum. Hydroceles can be secondarily infected. There are two subtypes of congenital hydrocele.
1. Encysted type with no communication with the peritoneum or tunica vaginalis, also called spermatic cord cyst. An encysted hydrocele is enclosed between two constrictions at the deep inguinal ring, just above the testis. It does not communicate with the peritoneum. It may be located anywhere along the spermatic cord and can be of any size or shape, but it does not change with increased peritoneal pressure. On ultrasound, an ovoid or round mass is seen in the groin along the spermatic cord; internal echogenicity varies depending on the content.
2. Funicular type which communicates with the peritoneum at the internal ring and does not surround the testis. This type is also called funiculocele. They are more frequently encountered in premature infant and children.

CASE 81

Testicular Trauma

CASE

A 40-year-old male with history of road traffic accident came to radiology department for CT scan.

Radiological Findings on CT Examination

Axial CT pelvis (Fig. 1) shows disrupted right testis and fluid collection in right scrotal sac suggestive of hematocele.

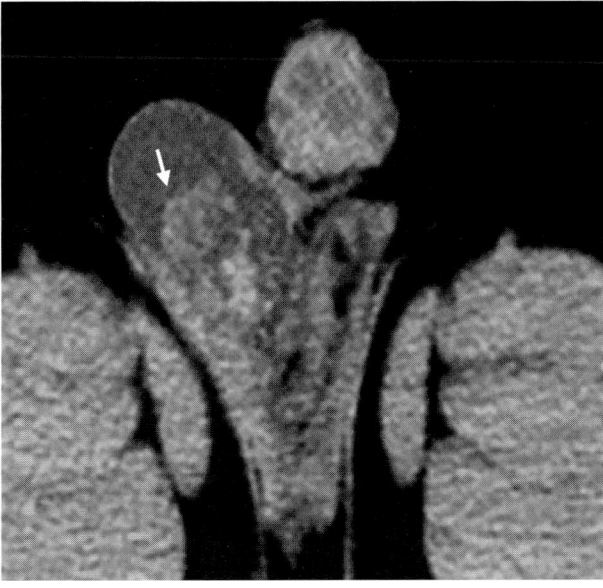

Fig. 1

Comments and Explanation

In trauma there is either a hematocele or testicular hematoma. In the acute phase the hemorrhage is hyperdense and in the chronic phase it is hypodense. A hematocele results from scrotal or intra-abdominal hemorrhage. It represents bleeding between the leaves of the tunica vaginalis and appears as a complex fluid collection. With time, this collection can develop loculations, which appear as thick septations. It is important to tell if the testis is intact, because if there is a rupture, this can sometimes be treated surgically. Testicular rupture is seen as focal alterations of testicular architecture. A discrete fracture plane is identified in fewer than 20% of cases, although visible alterations in the testicular contour are a common finding. The axial CT pelvis demonstrated a large hematocele.

Opinion

Testicular rupture with hematocele.

Clinical Discussion

Blunt injury (e.g. from an athletic accident or motor vehicle collision) is the most common cause of scrotal trauma, followed by penetrating injury from gunshot or other assault. Knowledge of the scrotal anatomy and appropriate imaging techniques are key for accurate evaluation of scrotal injuries. Ultrasonography (USG) is the first-line imaging modality to help guide therapy for scrotal trauma, except in degloving injury, which results in scrotal skin avulsion. Trauma often may result in hematoma, hydrocele, hematocele, testicular fracture, or testicular rupture. The timely diagnosis of rupture, based on a US finding of discontinuity of the echogenic tunica albuginea, is critical because emergent surgery results in salvage of the testis in 80–90% of rupture cases. The radiologist should be familiar also with other nuances associated with penetrating trauma, iatrogenic and postoperative complications, and electrical injury. Color flow and duplex Doppler imaging are highly useful techniques not only for assessing testicular viability and perfusion but also for evaluating associated vascular injuries such as pseudoaneurysms. Testicular torsion can occur as a result of minor/incidental trauma. Testicular torsion occurs when a testicle torts on the spermatic cord resulting in the cutting off of blood supply. Ultrasound is helpful in confirming the diagnosis. Testicular torsion implies obstruction of first venous, and later, arterial flow. The extent of testicular ischemia will depend on the degree of twisting (180°–720°) and the duration of the torsion. Key findings of a torsed testis on USG include twisting of the spermatic cord resulting in whirlpool sign which may be appreciated on Doppler and increase in size of the testis and epididymis. Homogeneous echotexture is an early finding, prior to necrosis. Heterogeneous echotexture is a late finding (after 24 hours), implies necrosis. The key to successful treatment is rapid diagnosis and surgical intervention. If diagnosed early enough the testis can be detorted with little damage. If the testis has necrosed, then orchidectomy is required.

CASE 82

Seminoma

CASE

A 28-year-old male with painless progressive swelling in left testis came for CT abdomen and pelvis.

Radiological Findings on CT Examination

Axial CT abdomen and pelvis shows a solid enhancing left testicular mass (Fig. 1A) and intra-abdominal lymphadenopathy (Fig. 1B).

Comments and Explanation

Abdominal and pelvic CT is important in visualizing metastases both as a part of primary staging of seminoma testes and also in primary diagnosis when a testicular mass is of unknown etiology. Metastases to the para-aortic lymph nodes at the level of the renal vessels are the typical first site of spread owing to the lymphatic drainage of the testicles relating to embryological testicular descent. The nodal metastases are often bulky, of homogeneous density and tend to encase surrounding vessels. Inguinal or iliac lymph node metastases suggest lymphatic spread via the scrotum and therefore local tumor extension beyond the tunica vaginalis. Visceral metastases are seen in around 5% of patients at presentation (lung, liver, bone, brain). Staging CT of the chest is only indicated when there is an abnormal chest X-ray. Fluoro-2-deoxy-D-glucose (FDG) positron emission tomography (PET) has been evaluated for its utility in staging and restaging of seminomatous and nonseminomatous tumors.

Opinion

Left testicular seminoma.

Section 18: Scrotum

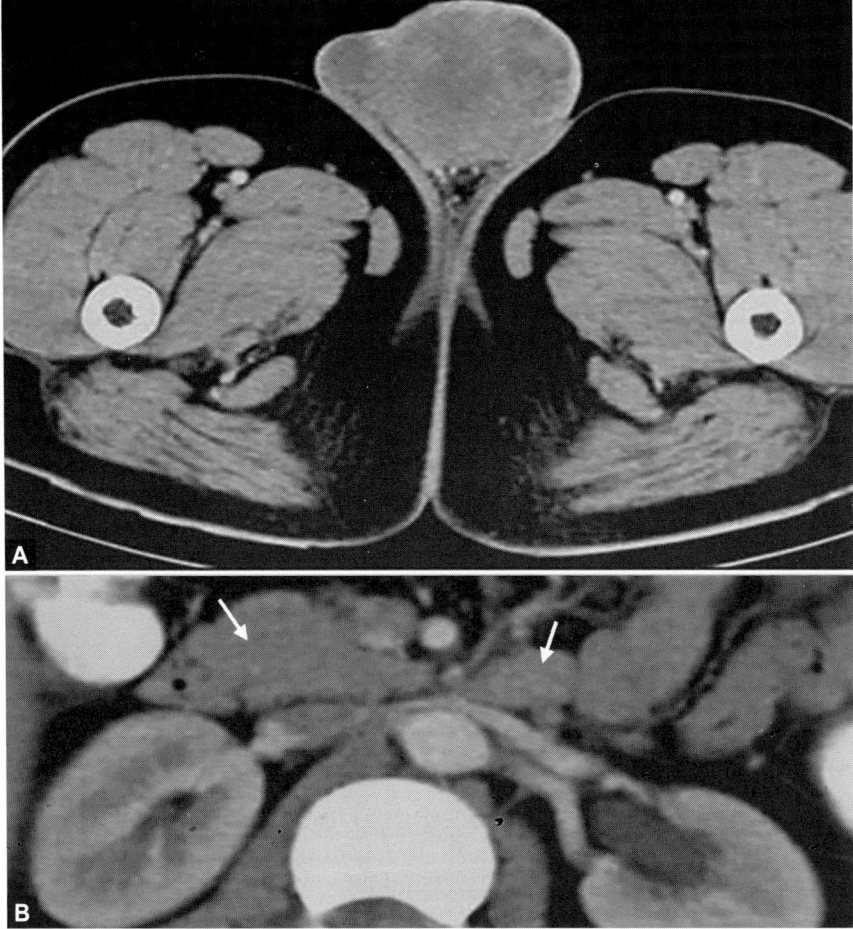

Figs 1A and B

Clinical Discussion

Germ cell tumors are the most common malignancy in men aged 15–35 years, with seminoma accounting for one third of such cases. Risk factors for seminoma are (1) Undescended testis is the major risk factor for testicular germ cell tumors; (2) Increased risk in the contralateral normally descended testis; (3) Previous tumor in contra lateral testis; (4) Family history of testicular germ cell tumor; (5) Testicular microlithiasis; (6) Other risk factors include infections such as HIV, mumps, orchitis and history of trauma or organ transplant immunosuppression. The most common presentation is with a painless testicular mass. Bilateral tumors are rare. Diagnosis following trauma is common as it draws the patient's attention to the lump. Back pain, abdominal discomfort or abdominal mass may be a presenting feature in the patients who have retroperitoneal nodal metastases. Presentation with distant and extra nodal metastases is rare.

CASE 83

Undescended Testis

CASE

A 6-year-old male child with empty scrotal sac was subjected to ultrasound and CT abdomen.

Radiological Findings on CT Examination

Ultrasound (Figs 1A and B) and CT abdomen and pelvis (Figs 1C and D) show right and left testis in respective inguinal regions suggestive of bilateral undescended testes.

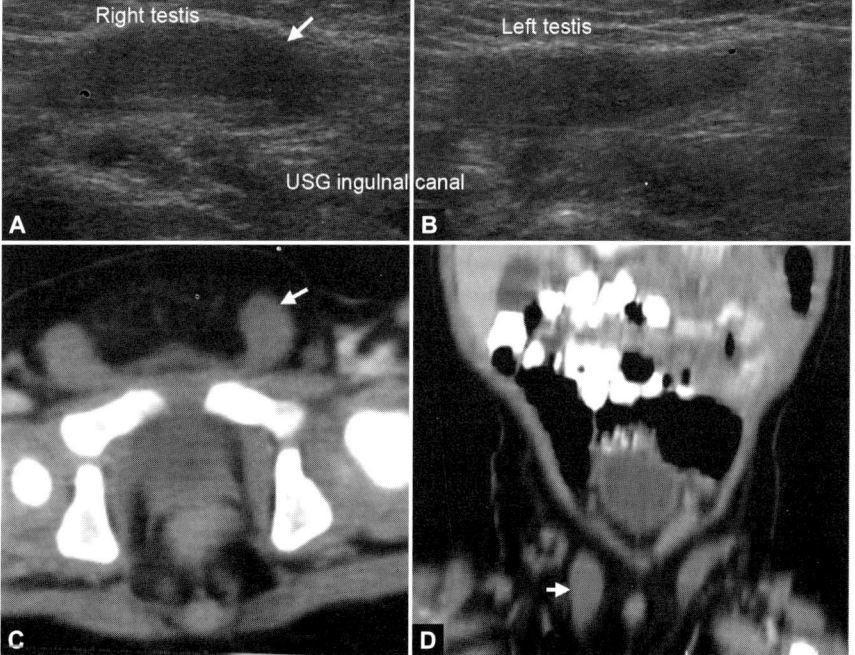

Figs 1A to D

Comments and Explanation

An absence of testes in the scrotal sac is called cryptorchidism and may be termed as undescended testes, ectopic testes, atrophic or absent testes. Ultrasound shows a homogeneously hypoechoic ovoid structure, similar to contralateral testes, with an echogenic mediastinum testes. Sonography is excellent in location of testes, high up in scrotum or within inguinal canal. However, its use is limited in intra-abdominal, pelvic or retroperitoneal/ectopic testes. Ultrasound is also inconclusive in atrophic small testes, where it is difficult to differentiate from lymph nodes. MRI is the best cross-sectional modality to assess cryptorchidism. Coronal T1W images can show gubernaculum testes and spermatic cord, which can be followed to locate the undescended testes. Also, ectopic pelvic or retroperitoneal location of testes can be identified. Diffusion-weighted MRI shows restriction and hyperintense testes.

Opinion

Undescended testes.

Clinical Discussion

Testes remain in the intra-abdominal location till 7 months of gestation, when it descends into the inguinal canal through the deep inguinal ring. The gubernaculum is the ligament, which connects the testes to the scrotum. Under hormonal influence gubernaculum testes contracts, and testes descends into the scrotum. Undescended testes are associated with premature birth, smoking and alcohol intake during pregnancy, androgen, Prader-Willi syndrome, Noonan syndrome, cloacal exstrophy, Prune-Belly syndrome and gestational diabetes.

Orchidopexy is the preferred procedure in case of viable testes high-up in scrotum or within inguinal canal. However, it is done after 1 year of age because testes may descend during first year of life under testosterone influence. Any nonviable, atrophic or ectopic testis is however not left, and orchidectomy is the only option as there is high risk of malignant transformation.

SECTION 19

Penis

84. Penile Carcinoma

CASE 84

Penile Carcinoma

CASE

A 56-year-old male with history of foul smelling discharge from penis with sore came to department of radiology for CT abdomen and pelvis.

Radiological Findings on CT Examination

CT pelvis is showing enhancing mass and architectural distortion of glans and extending to the shaft of penis (Figs 1A and B).

Comments and Explanation

Squamous cell carcinoma of the penis is most commonly located in the glans penis in 40% of cases. In decreasing order of frequency, other locations include the prepuce, coronal sulcus, and shaft. The spread of penile cancer usually

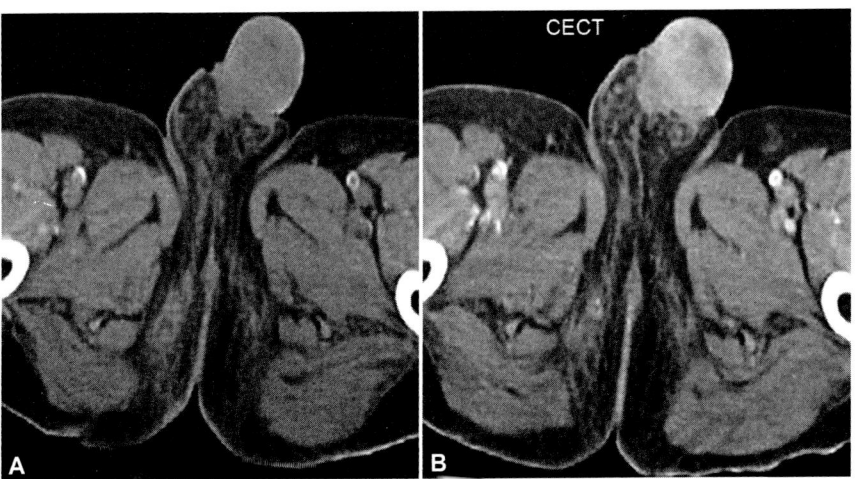

Figs 1A and B

occurs via lymphatic vessels, with the Buck fascia acting as a barrier to corporal invasion and hematogenous spread. The lymphatic spread of cancer from the penis differs with the location of the primary lesion. The lymphatic vessels of the skin of the penis and prepuce drain primarily into the superficial inguinal nodes. The lymphatic vessels of the glans penis drain into the deep inguinal and external iliac nodes, and those of the erectile tissue and penile urethra drain into the internal iliac nodes. Because there is communication between lymphatic vessels, bilateral lymphadenopathy may be seen with a unilateral tumor. Invariably, the lymphatic vessels of the penis first drain into the inguinal nodes before reaching the pelvic nodes.

Opinion

Penile carcinoma.

Clinical Discussion

Patients with penile carcinoma presents with complaints of redness, rash and foul smelling discharge from the penis, pain, growth or sore on the penis of more than four weeks duration, generally occurs above 55 years of age, bleeding from the penis or from under the fore skin, change in color of the penis or phimosis. Risk factors for penile carcinoma include HIV, human papillomavirus (HPV), genital warts, poor hygiene, smegma, balanitis, phimosis, and paraphimosis. The treatment of penile cancer varies depending on the site and extent of the primary cancer and the presence of metastatic inguinal lymphadenopathy. Circumcision alone may cure patients with small tumors of the distal prepuce, whereas tumors of the glans penis and distal shaft require partial penectomy, including a 2-cm tumor-free margin. Bulky tumors of the proximal penis are treated with total penectomy and perineal urethrostomy. Inguinal lymphadenectomy can be performed at the time of the penile surgery or later. The current approach for dealing with palpable inguinal lymph nodes includes re-evaluation after 4-6 weeks of antibiotic therapy. This approach is based on the principle that reactive lymphadenopathy will resolve following antibiotic treatment, whereas neoplastic lymphadenopathy will persist. The continued presence of lymph nodes in the inguinal region is treated with bilateral inguinal lymphadenectomy. Radiation therapy with external beam irradiation and brachytherapy has yielded local control rates similar to those for surgical resection. Radiation therapy and laser therapy are the best conservative therapeutic options for localized disease. Treatment for metastases is generally palliative.

SECTION 20

Uterus

85. Broad Ligament Fibroid
86. Hydrometrocolpos
87. Pyometra
88. Endometrial Carcinoma
89. Carcinoma Cervix
90. Vaginal Carcinoma
91. Ureterovaginal Fistula
92. Vulval Carcinoma

CASE 85

Broad Ligament Fibroid

CASE

A 35-year-old female with history of pain in lower abdomen was referred to radiology department for CT scan abdomen including pelvis.

Radiological Findings on CT Examination

CT shows a homogeneous moderately enhancing well defined soft tissue density mass in left adnexa (F) attached to superolateral aspect of uterus (U). Left ovary is seen separately from the mass (O). It has same imaging characteristics as the uterine myometrium (Figs 1A to D). Findings are suggestive of broad ligament fibroid.

Comments and Explanation

A broad ligament fibroid occurs in relation to the broad ligament and is considered as variation of uterine leiomyoma. Usually seen as hypoechoic, solid, well-circumscribed adnexal mass, larger lesions show heterogeneous appearance. There is no interface between tumor and uterus and no relation to the ipsilateral ovary. CT imaging characteristics are similar to uterine fibroid. They are usually of soft tissue density but may exhibit coarse peripheral or central calcification with variable enhancement pattern. On MRI signal characteristics in uncomplicated cases are essentially similar to a uterine leiomyoma. Fibroids appear as sharply marginated areas of low to intermediate signal intensity on T1- and T2-weighted MRI scans. Most lesions enhance on post contrast images similarly to the myometrium, while larger leiomyomas tend to enhance heterogeneously.

Opinion

Broad ligament fibroid.

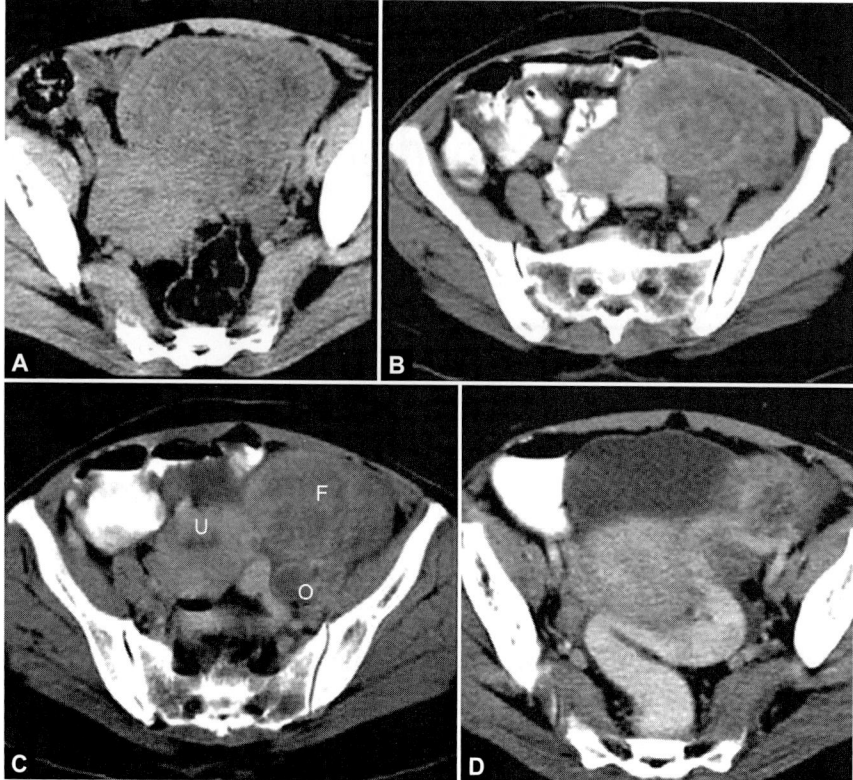

Figs 1A to D

Clinical Discussion

It is an extra-uterine leiomyoma arising from the broad ligament usually from a stalk. Torsion of the leiomyoma can occur if it is pedunculated. Differential diagnosis include unusual leiomyomas like pedunculated sub-serosal leiomyoma projecting towards the broad ligament, solid ovarian neoplasms particularly those with dominant fibrous components like ovarian fibroma, fibrothecoma and Brenner tumor which are inseparable from the ovary.

CASE

86 Hydrometrocolpos

CASE

A 11-year-old patient came with history of pain in abdomen since 5 days and was referred to radiology department for CT scan abdomen.

Radiological Findings on CT Scan

CT scan pelvis shows a large well defined elliptical collection seen in the uterine endometrial cavity and also in vagina (Figs 1A to D). The contents of this collection are clear.

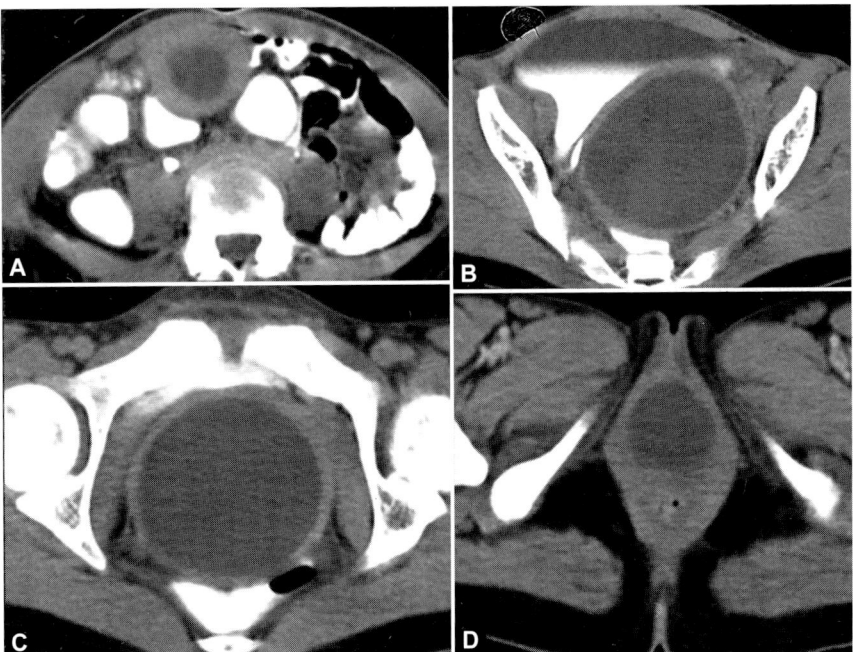

Figs 1A to D

Comments and Explanation

Hydro/hematometrocolpos is accumulation of sterile fluid (hydro)/blood (hemato)/or pus (pyo) within the uterus (metra) and vagina (colpos). The condition is caused by an obstruction due to an imperforate hymen, a transverse vaginal septum, or stenosis-atresia of the vagina. Presents either in infancy (due to influence of maternal hormones) or puberty. Vagina usually dilates more than uterus (due to elastic walls) and are associated with Müllerian duct anomalies (especially didelphys uterus). Sonographically, there is a cystic midline mass that may contain mildly echogenic areas in the fluid collection representing mucous secretions or blood. CT can also show distended fluid filled uterine cavity and vagina. MR is sometimes helpful for further evaluation, especially if Müllerian duct anomaly is present. Associated abnormalities are uterine didelphys, bicornuate uterus, renal agenesis, intestinal aganglionosis, imperforate anus, urogenital sinus and also vertebral and cardiac anomalies.

Opinion

Hydrometrocolpos.

Clinical Discussion

Hydrometrocolpos is characterized by an expanded fluid filled vaginal cavity with associated distention of the uterine cavity. It may present in infancy with a lower abdominal mass, or be delayed till menarche. Hydrocolpos and hydrometrocolpos are due to vaginal or cervical obstruction and can present in either the newborn period or around puberty. In newborn girls, hydrometrocolpos accounts for 15% of abdominal masses. Obstructions caused by an imperforate hymen are generally not associated with other congenital abnormalities. Frequently, imperforate anus, cloacal exstrophy, and persistent urogenital sinus will have associated hydrometrocolpos. McKusick-Kaufman syndrome is an autosomal recessive multiple malformation syndrome characterized by hydrometrocolpos and postaxial polydactyly. Mayer-Rokitansky-Küster-Hauser syndrome combines a variety of uterine anomalies, vaginal atresia with normal Fallopian tubes and ovaries, and is the second most common cause of primary amenorrhea. Complications of hydrometrocolpos include reflux of the endometrial tissue via the Fallopian tubes (i.e. hematosalpinx) may result in secondary endometriosis, endo-/myo-/parametritis, hydronephrosis, pelvic abscess and urinary tract infection.

CASE
87
Pyometra

CASE

A 55-year-old female with history of carcinoma cervix and post chemotherapy came with a history of pain abdomen, fever and distension.

Radiological Findings on CT Scan Examination

Contrast-enhanced computed tomography (CECT) scan of pelvis (Figs 1A to D) shows enhancing large fluid collections in the uterus in a patient who had earlier

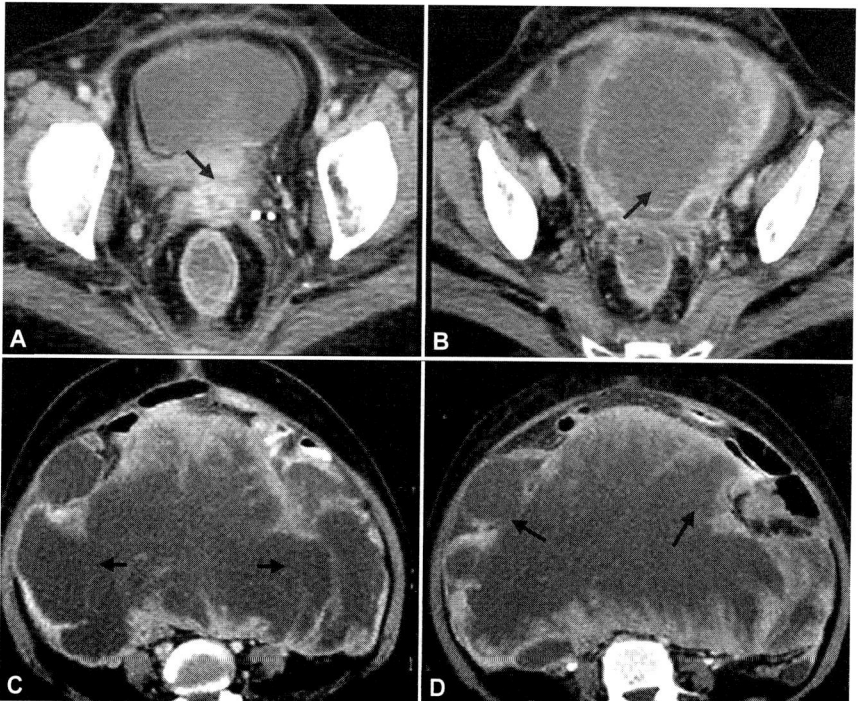

Figs 1A to D

undergone chemotherapy for carcinoma cervix. No mass is seen in the cervix however it is stenosed.

Comments and Explanation

Pyometra is an infection of endometrial cavity and a collection of pus distending the uterine cavity. It occurs principally when there is a stenosed cervical os, usually due to uterine or cervical malignancy. In order for pyometra to develop, there must be both an infection and blockage of cervix. Signs and symptoms include lower abdominal pain, fever with rigors, and discharge of pus from uterus.

Opinion

Pyometra.

Clinical Discussion

Causes of pyometra are endometritis/pelvic inflammatory disease, uterine malignancies, pelvic irradiation, cervical stenosis, retained products of conception, imperforate hymen. It is more common in postmenopausal women than women of child bearing age in whom hematometra is more common. CT shows enhancing collection in the uterine cavity. In case of ruptured pyometra CT shows evidence of ascites with features of inflammation. Exploratory laparotomy is diagnostic.

CASE 88

Endometrial Carcinoma

CASE

A 59-year-old female with history of post menopausal bleeding was referred to radiology department for CT scan abdomen and pelvis.

Radiological Findings on CT Examination

CT shows collection in the uterine cavity lined on all sides by a thick irregular endometrial wall (Figs 1A to D). Biopsy proved this to be a high grade carcinoma of endometrium.

Comments and Explanation

The diagnosis of endometrial carcinoma is usually made by endometrial biopsy or by dilatation and curettage. Transvaginal ultrasound is the preferred method of screening for endometrial abnormalities in high-risk patients such as those on estrogen replacement therapy and tamoxifen treatment for breast carcinoma. The appearance of endometrial carcinoma on ultrasound is variable, ranging from a completely normal-appearing uterus; to echogenic thickening of the endometrium (greater than 15 mm in premenopausal and greater than 5 mm in postmenopausal women); to an irregular, heterogeneous, hyperechoic endometrium with ill-defined hypoechoic or isoechoic areas. CT has a role in assessing for distant metastases. Although not generally used for initial diagnosis or local staging, endometrial carcinoma may be encountered on CT. Oral, rectal, and IV administration of contrast material is necessary for optimal CT evaluation. Following IV contrast administration, nonuniform contrast enhancement of the tumor may occur but to a much lesser degree than the usually intense and uniform enhancement of the normal myometrium. Thus, the endometrial tumor may become apparent on postcontrast images as a lesion with relatively low attenuation. On post contrast CT it may show diffuse thickening or mass within endometrial cavity. Endometrial carcinoma spreads by local infiltration from the endometrium to the myometrium and along the lower uterine segment to the cervix. Other routes of spread follow lymphatic channels.

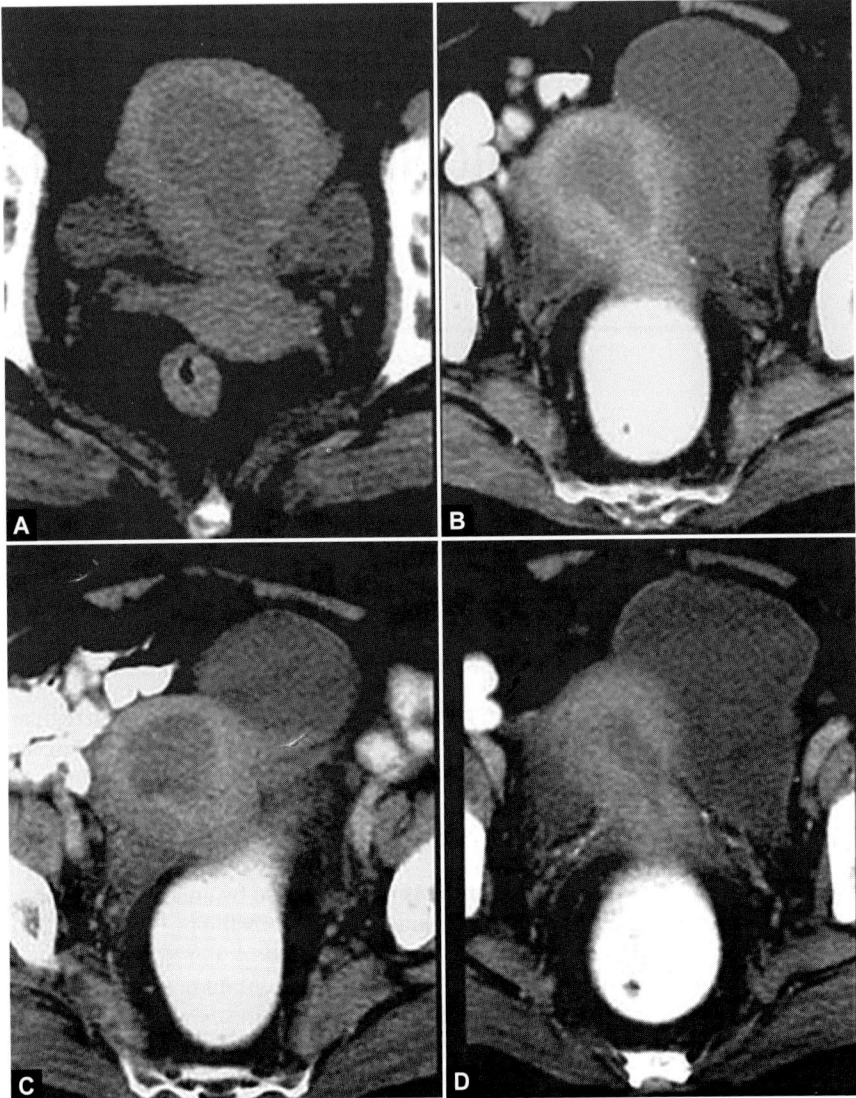

Figs 1A to D

Opinion

Endometrial carcinoma.

Clinical Discussion

Endometrial carcinoma is the most common gynecologic cancer. Risk factors include obesity, nulliparity, estrogen replacement, estrogen-secreting ovarian tumors, late-onset menopause, diabetes mellitus, anovulatory cycles, polycystic ovaries, and adenomatous hyperplasia. Most endometrial cancers are adenocarcinomas. Presentation peaks at around the 6th decade. Patients commonly present at an early stage, with post menopausal bleeding as the initial symptom. CT is the imaging modality used most commonly in clinical practice to determine the extent of spread of endometrial cancer. It can also present as polypoid mass surrounded by endometrial fluid or as a heterogeneous soft tissue mass and fluid expanding the endometrial cavity.

CT staging of endometrial cancer is based on the surgical/pathologic FIGO classification, as shown below:

Stage I: Tumor confined to the uterine corpus
Stage II: Tumor invades cervical stroma, but does not extend beyond the uterus
Stage III: Local and/or regional spread of the tumor
Stage IV: Tumor invades bladder and/or bowel mucosa and/or distant metastases.

CASE 89

Carcinoma Cervix

CASE

A 43-year-old female came with history of vaginal bleeding and discharge and was referred to radiology department for CT scan.

Radiological Findings on CT Examination

Figures 1A to E (A) Plain CT pelvis (Fig. 1A) shows a hyperdense cervical mass with loss of fat plane anteriorly with urinary bladder and posteriorly with rectum; (B) Immediate postcontrast CT shows normal contrast uptake by left kidney. Right kidney shows gross hydronephrosis; (C to E) show invasion of the uterus, urinary bladder, rectum and right lower ureter.

Comments and Explanation

In locally confined disease, a cervical mass may be seen by ultrasound. In locally advanced disease, the cervix may become diffusely enlarged, inhomogeneous, and irregularly marginated.

Cervical cancer and the normal cervical stroma usually have similar attenuations on CT images that are obtained without intravenous contrast enhancement. Therefore, the tumor and the normal cervical parenchyma cannot be reliably distinguished on nonenhanced CT scans. After the intravenous administration of contrast material CT shows an enlarged cervix with normal contrast enhancement or an enlarged cervix with inhomogeneous areas of hypoattenuation but without a discrete mass that is clearly delineated or an enlarged cervix with a circumscribed solid mass that has an enhancement which is less than that of the normal cervical stroma and shows a homogeneous or heterogeneous hypoattenuation. Cervical cancer frequently obstructs the endocervical canal, resulting in accumulation of serous, hemorrhagic, or purulent fluid in the uterine cavity. The presence of hydrometras should raise the suspicion of cervical or endometrial carcinoma. Cervical cancer spreads by either local infiltration into parametrium, pelvic sidewall, and adjacent organs (vagina, ureters, bladder, and rectum) or by lymphatic spread to the pelvic (obturator and

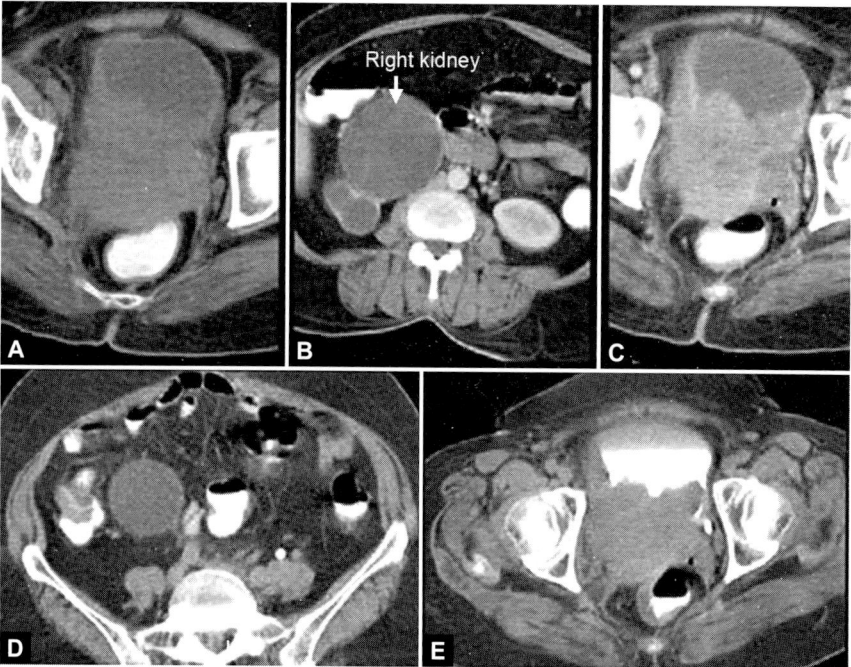

Figs 1A to E

external, internal, and common iliac) and para-aortic lymph node. In advanced cases hematogenous metastases to the lungs, liver, brain, and bones can occur.

Opinion

Carcinoma of cervix.

Clinical Discussion

Carcinoma of the cervix is a malignancy arising from the cervix. It typically presents in younger women with the average age of onset at around 45 years. Risk factors include human papilloma virus infection, multiple sexual partners and early age of first sexual intercourse. Cervical carcinoma arises from the squamo-columnar junction. In order to be radiographically visible, tumors must be at least stage Ib or above. MRI is the imaging modality of choice to depict the primary tumor and assess local extent due to its improved contrast resolution and multiplanar capability. Distant metastatic disease is best assessed with CT or PET where available. CT in general is not very useful in assessment of the primary tumor but can be useful in assessing advanced disease. It is performed primarily to assess adenopathy but also has roles in defining advanced disease, monitoring distant metastasis, planning the placement of radiation ports, and guiding percutaneous biopsy. The treatment and prognosis of invasive cervical carcinoma depends on tumor volume, extent of disease, histological grade, vascular and lymphatic spread.

CASE 90

Vaginal Carcinoma

CASE

A 55-year-old female with complaints of pain in pelvis and vaginal bleeding was referred for CT abdomen and pelvis.

Radiological Findings on CT Examination

Contrast-enhanced computed tomography (CECT) scan abdomen and pelvis (Figs 1A and B) shows abnormal enhancing soft tissue seen in the region of the vault and entire vagina with few nonenhancing necrotic areas. The lesion is seen abutting the rectum with loss of fat planes and is also seen involving the anal canal. Bilateral iliac and right inguinal lymphadenopathy are also seen.

Comments and Explanation

Squamous cell carcinoma makes up about 85% of primary vaginal malignancies. This tumor arises from the posterior wall of the upper third of the vagina. The main patterns of disease are an ulcerating or fungating mass or an annular constricting lesion. CT is recommended for assessment of groin, pelvis, and extra pelvic lymph

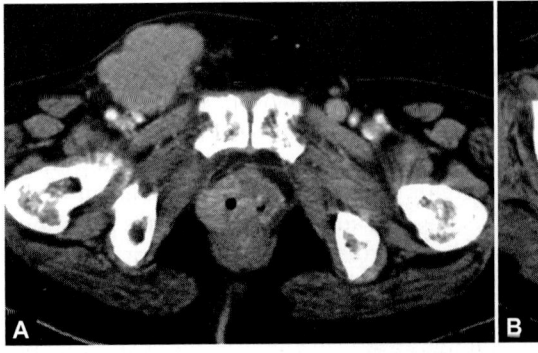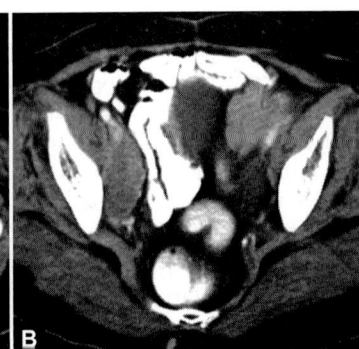

Figs 1A and B

node metastasis. CT criteria for lymph node metastases are based on short-axis diameter of ≥ 1 cm, thus, CT cannot detect metastases in lymph nodes < 1 cm. Because the treatment and prognosis change with the presence of pelvic lymph node metastases, it is imperative to find the metastases. CT is not helpful in local staging of the tumor because of its low soft-tissue contrast resolution; however, CT can assess the involvement of bladder or the rectum, detect metastases to the lungs and the bone, and help plan radiation treatment. At magnetic resonance (MR) imaging, squamous cell carcinoma has intermediate signal intensity on T2-weighted images and low signal intensity on T1-weighted images.

Opinion

Vaginal carcinoma with lymph node metastasis.

Clinical Discussion

Carcinoma *in situ* is often treated with surgery. However, the standard therapeutic intervention for patients with carcinoma of the vagina is radiation therapy. Advanced stages are often treated with radiotherapy and chemotherapy.

CASE 91

Ureterovaginal Fistula

CASE

A 50-year-old female with history of hysterectomy 7 months back complaining of urinary incontinence through vagina was referred to radiology department for CT scan abdomen and pelvis.

Radiological Findings on CT Examination

Early post contrast CT image of pelvis shows fluid in vagina (Fig. 1A). The vagina is completely opacified with contrast on delayed image (Fig. 1B). Hydronephrosis and hydroureter is seen on left side. The left distal ureter is communicating with the vagina (Fig. 1C) as a result of ureterovaginal fistula.

Comments and Explanation

Uretero-vaginal fistula refers to a fistulous communication between ureter and vagina. The diagnosis may be made by direct visualization on vaginoscopy and cystourethroscopy. Excretory urography can help in diagnosing ureterovaginal fistula. In this a vaginal swab is kept during the procedure, which gets soaked with contrast. Although, differentiation with vesicovaginal fistula is difficult, oblique images may demonstrate ureterovaginal fistula. Delayed contrast enhanced CT helps in direct visualization of the fistulous tract. Vesicovaginal fistula may be a co-existing finding.

Opinion

Ureterovaginal fistula.

Clinical Discussion

Patients of ureterovaginal fistula come with complaints of incontinence of urine, fever with chills due to secondary urinary tract infections. Ureterovaginal fistula predominantly occurs as a result of ureteral injury during gynecological/

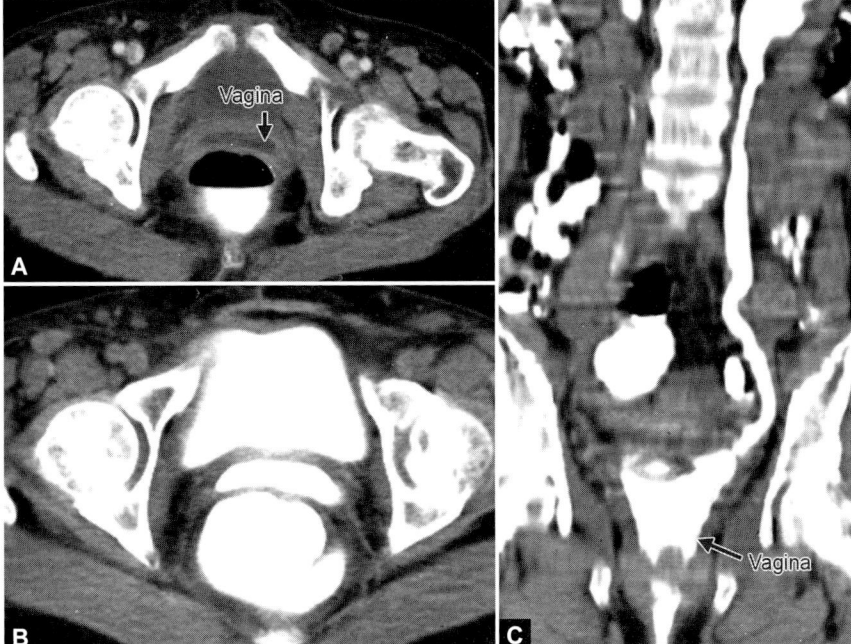

Figs 1A to C

obstetric surgery like abdominal/vaginal/radical hysterectomy, cesarean section and other pelvic surgical procedures like vascular and urological surgery. This fistula can also result from locally advanced malignant disease, radiation therapy and pelvic trauma. The main aim of the treatment of ureterovaginal fistula is the resolution of the urinary leakage, prevention of urosepsis and preservation of renal function. Treatment of choice is nephrostomy and ureteral stent placement. Complications associated with ureterovaginal fistula repair, are urinary extravasation and ureteral stricture formation.

CASE 92

Vulval Carcinoma

CASE

A 75-year-old female came with history of vaginal growth and bleeding. CT abdomen and pelvis was done.

Radiological Findings on CT Scan Examination

Figure 1 shows asymmetric soft tissue density lesion seen in vulva on right side. No local or distant intra-abdominal metastases were seen on contrast CT abdomen. Biopsy showed it to be a squamous cell carcinoma of vulva.

Comments and explanation

Primary vulvar cancer is a rare gynecological malignancy that originates from the vulva. The most common histological type by far is squamous cell carcinoma.

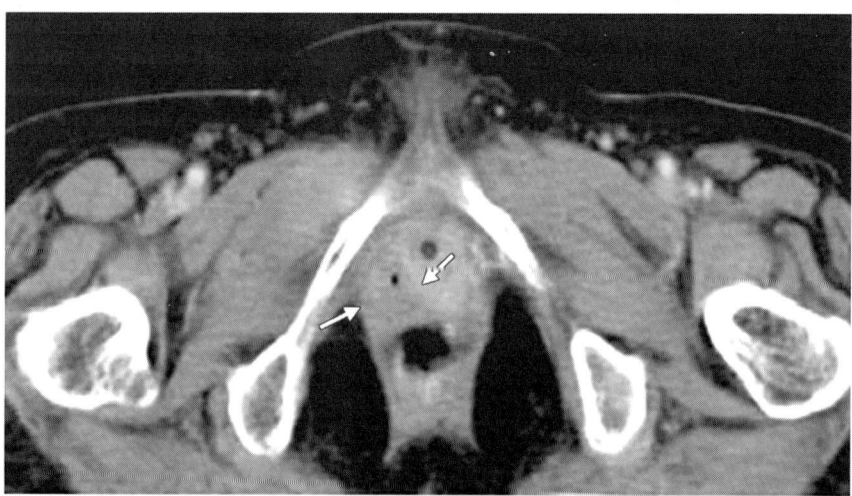

Fig. 1

The tumor commonly involves the labia majora and minora. The labia majora are the most common site followed by the labia minora. The clitoris may rarely be involved. CT scan gives information about the size, shape, and position of tumors and can be helpful to see if the cancer has spread to other organs. It can also help find enlarged lymph nodes. MRI is useful in accurately assessing the size of vulval lesion and assessing groin lymph node metastasis. Overall, MRI may be best suited for determining the extent of local disease and invasion, although it is also helpful in identifying groin nodal metastases and assessing the depth of these nodes from the skin, which assist radiation planning. CT and PET/CT can help detect and determine the extent of distant disease, however, PET/CT is best used to identify lymph node metastases, where clinical assessment fails and detect distant spread, which ultimately supports optimal treatment planning.

Opinion

Vulval carcinoma.

Clinical Discussion

The cause of vulvar cancer is unclear; however, some conditions such as lichen sclerosus, squamous dysplasia or chronic vulvar itching may precede cancer. In younger women affected with vulval cancer, risk factors include low socioeconomic status, human papillomavirus (HPV) infection, multiple sexual partners, cigarette use and cervical cancer. Patients that are infected with HIV tend to be more susceptible to vulvar cancer as well. Typically, a lesion presents in the form of a lump or ulcer and may be associated with itching, irritation, local bleeding or discharge or pain during sexual intercourse. Adenocarcinoma can arise from the bartholin gland and present with a painful lump. MRI may play a role in evaluation of the local extent of disease in advanced cases, especially if urethral invasion is suspected, as well as in the evaluation of lymphadenopathy. Vulval cancer appears on US as a soft-tissue mass with internal vascularity. On CT, vulval cancer appears as a nonspecific soft-tissue mass. On MRI, it demonstrates intermediate signal intensity on T1W sequences and high signal intensity on T2W sequences. MRI may also be used to differentiate recurrence from post-therapy changes.

SECTION 21

Ovary

93. Ovarian Vein Thrombosis
94. Ovarian Tumor

CASE 93

Ovarian Vein Thrombosis

CASE

A 26-year-old postpartum female came with history of lower abdominal pain and fever not responding to antibiotics and was referred to department of radiology for CT abdomen and pelvis.

Radiological Findings on CT Examination

CECT pelvis (Fig. 1) shows intravascular filling defects in both ovarian veins diagnosed as bilateral ovarian vein thrombosis.

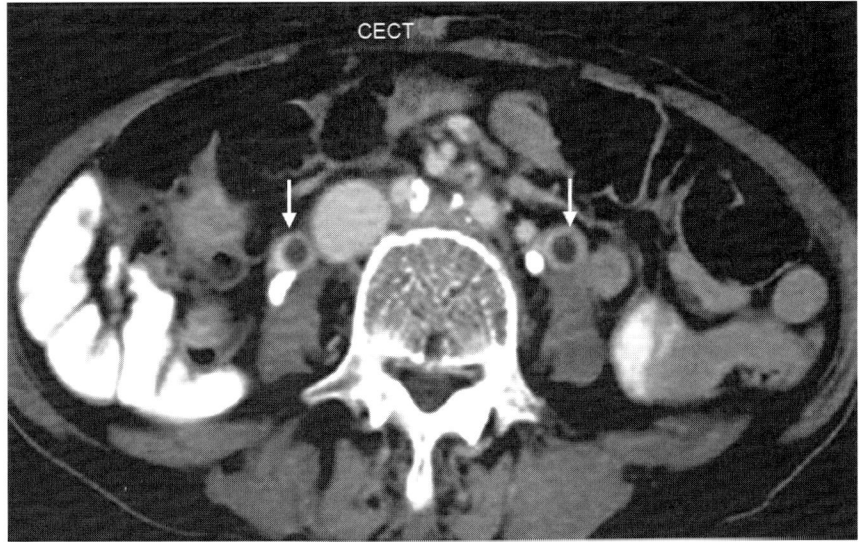

Fig. 1

Comments and Explanation

Ovarian vein thrombosis (OVT) occurs most commonly in postpartum patients, and can result in pulmonary emboli. Presentation is usually with acute pelvic pain in the post partum period, where it is termed puerperal ovarian vein thrombosis (POVT) or post-partum ovarian vein thrombosis. On sonography, the thrombosed ovarian vein appears as an anechoic to hypoechoic tubular structure extending superiorly from the adnexa, lateral to the IVC or aorta retroperitoneally. Doppler ultrasound can provide a quick and inexpensive initial examination with findings of absence of color-flow filling and spectral waveform. CT angiography is the investigation of choice. On CECT the thrombosed ovarian vein is visualized as an enlarged tubular retroperitoneal structure, originating in the region of the adnexa and extending cephalad in the retroperitoneal region to the level of the renal veins, representing thrombus with peripheral rim-enhancement of the vein. Secondary signs on CT scans are perivascular inflammatory stranding, an enlarged uterus that contains fluid, and inhomogeneously enhancing parauterine mass believed to be secondary to accompanying pelvic thrombophlebitis. Multiplanar reconstructed coronal images would improve visualization of the IVC thrombus in its entire length, therefore are helpful in evaluating the extent of a thrombus.

Opinion

Bilateral ovarian vein thrombosis.

Clinical Discussion

Postpartum ovarian vein thrombosis is an uncommon complication of the postpartum period. OVT can be accurately diagnosed by appropriate noninvasive radiologic modalities to start early therapy with anticoagulants and intravenous antibiotics. OVT can cause serious complications such as sepsis, IVC thrombosis, pulmonary thromboembolism, and renal vein thrombosis and they may cause death. OVT occurs 80–90% on the right side; this could be caused by compression of the right ovarian vein against the sacral promontory due to an enlarged retroverted uterus and presence of retrograde flow in the left ovarian vein. Most commonly the right ovarian vein is involved, possibly due to retrograde flow in the left vein preventing stasis and ascending infection. The CT findings consist of a tubular structure with an enhancing wall and low-attenuation thrombus in the ovarian veins. In patients in whom ultrasound examination is suboptimal, due to overlying bowel gas, MRI should be preferred over CT because it does not require intravenous administration of iodinated contrast material and has no risk of radiation, and allows optimal evaluation of the inferior vena cava.

CASE 94

Ovarian Tumor

CASE

A 65-year-old female came with history of pain and lump in abdomen and was referred to radiology department for CT scan abdomen and pelvis.

Radiological Findings on CT Examination

CT abdomen and pelvis shows a moderately enhancing soft tissue density lesion in right adnexa. Right ovary is not seen separately from the mass. This turned out to be an undifferentiated epithelial ovarian malignancy (Figs 1A and B).

In another case contrast CT abdomen shows a large cystic lesion with enhancing thick septae and enhancing mural nodules arising from right ovary confirmed as adenocarcinoma (Figs 2A to D).

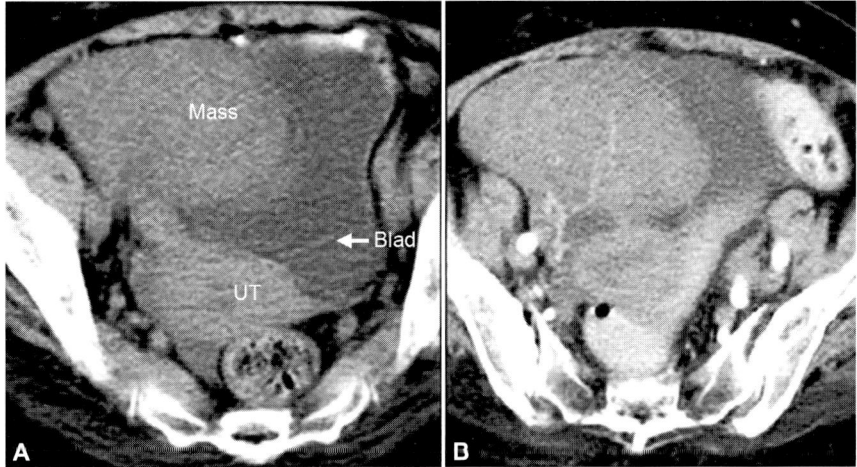

Figs 1A and B

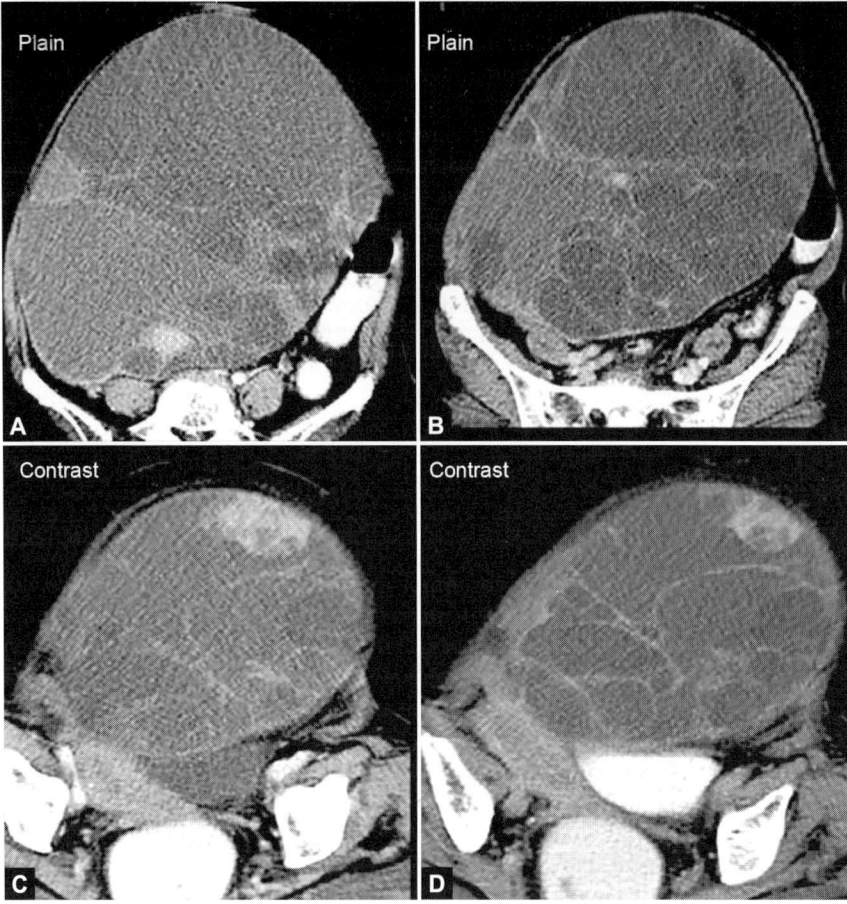

Figs 2A to D

Comments and Explanation

The imaging appearance of ovarian tumors ranges from cystic to solid masses. Epithelial ovarian tumors represent 60% of all ovarian neoplasms and 85% of malignant ovarian neoplasms. Subtypes of epithelial tumors include serous, mucinous, endometrioid, clear cell, and Brenner tumors. Serous cystadenoma is a thin-walled, unilocular or multilocular tumor filled with serous fluid. This tumor is very common and may mimic a physiologic cyst or, occasionally, an atypical mature cystic teratoma that lacks the characteristic eccentric mural nodule. Mucinous cystadenoma is less common, is almost always multilocular, and may be large. In many of these tumors, the MR imaging and CT appearance of the individual locules may vary as a result of differences in degree of hemorrhage or protein content. Although there is considerable overlap in morphologic characteristics and corresponding imaging features that in many cases prevents definitive preoperative characterization as benign or malignant. Features that are suggestive of malignant epithelial tumors include a thick, irregular wall; thick septae; papillary projections; and a large soft-tissue component with necrosis.

Opinion

Ovarian tumor.

Clinical Discussion

Ovarian tumors are classified as epithelial tumors, germ cell tumors, sex cord–stromal cell tumors, and metastatic tumors on the basis of tumor origin. Characterization of an ovarian mass is of the utmost importance in the preoperative evaluation of an ovarian neoplasm. It helps in deciding the management. Epithelial ovarian tumors can be classified as benign, malignant or borderline. The two most common types of epithelial neoplasms are serous and mucinous tumors. A benign serous cystadenoma manifests as a unilocular or multilocular cystic mass with homogeneous CT attenuation, a thin regular wall or septum, and no endocystic or exocystic vegetation. A tumor that manifests as a multilocular cystic mass that has a thin regular wall and septa or which has liquids of different attenuation but has no endocystic or exocystic vegetation is considered to be a benign mucinous cystadenoma. Mucinous cystadenomas tend to be larger than serous cystadenomas at presentation. Bilaterality and peritoneal carcinomatosis are seen more frequently in serous than in mucinous cystadenocarcinomas. Mucinous adenocarcinoma can rupture and is associated with pseudomyxoma peritonei. Features that are more suggestive of benign epithelial tumors include a diameter less than 4 cm, entirely cystic components, a wall thickness less than 3 mm, lack of internal structure, and the absence of both ascites and invasive characteristics such as peritoneal disease or adenopathy. Imaging findings that are suggestive of malignant tumors include a thick, irregular wall; thick septa; papillary projections; and a large soft-tissue component with necrosis. Ancillary findings include pelvic organ invasion, and implants (peritoneal, omental, mesenteric), ascites, and adenopathy increase diagnostic confidence for malignancy. Features such as wall thickening, septa, and multilocularity are less reliable indicators of malignancy because they are frequently seen in benign neoplasms, particularly cystadenofibromas, mucinous cystadenomas, and endometriomas. Mature teratoma is the most common benign ovarian tumor in women less than 45 years old. At CT, fat attenuation within a cyst, with or without calcification in the wall, is diagnostic for mature cystic teratoma. Benign ovarian enlargement includes mature cystic teratomas, cystadenomas and fibrothecomas. Mature cystic teratoma may be associated with complications from torsion, rupture, or malignant degeneration. Bilateral solid ovarian enlargement may be benign or malignant.

SECTION 22

Abdominal Wall

95. Abdominal Wall Sarcoma
96. Abdominal Wall Hernia

CASE

95 Abdominal Wall Sarcoma

CASE

A 70-year-old male with history of abdominal distension and loss of weight was referred to the department of radiology for CT scan abdomen.

Radiological Findings on CT Examination

Axial post contrast CT image of abdomen (Fig. 1) shows a large heterogeneous soft tissue mass seen to arise from the anterior abdominal wall. The lesion is

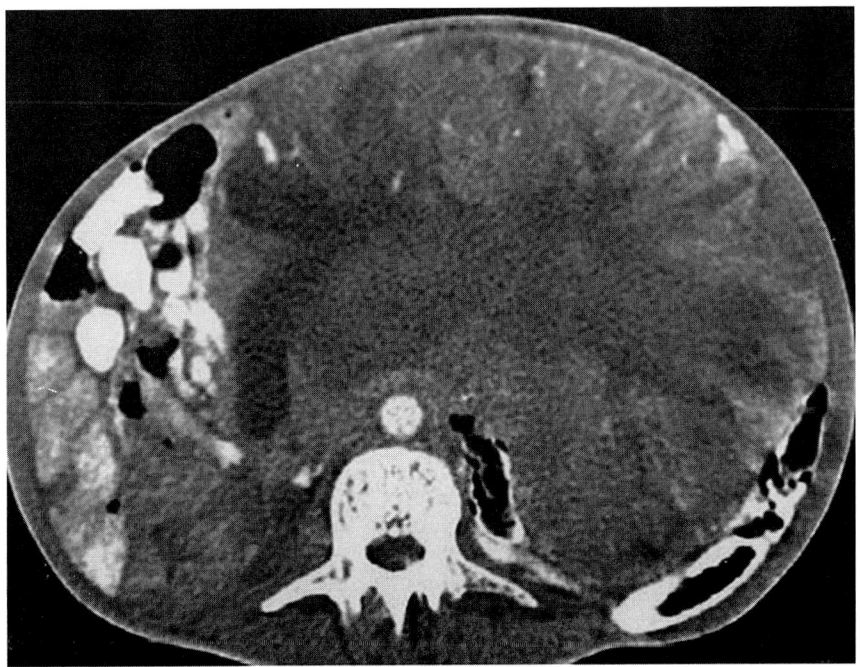

Fig. 1

having central hypodense areas and peripheral enhancement. The bowel loops are displaced posteriorly and laterally. There is no evidence of calcification within the lesion. On histopathological examination it turned out to be abdominal sarcoma.

Comments and Explanation

Sarcoma is malignant tumor of mesenchymal origin, that originates from the soft tissues rather than bone. They are classified on the basis of tissue seen on histology. Soft-tissue sarcomas are rare tumors that can affect any age, gender, and anatomic subsite. They have unique growth features, tending to extend within compartments and along fascial planes on a path of least resistance. On CT sarcomas are predominantly large, poorly demarcated, heterogeneous masses of muscle density with hemorrhage or necrosis. Computed tomography is useful for detection, defining extent, and predicting resectability of the primary tumor, evaluation of response to treatment, and detecting recurrence and metastasis.

Opinion

Abdominal wall sarcoma.

Clinical Discussion

A mass is the most common sign of a soft tissue tumor. It usually is painless. It grows through the lines of least resistance so symptoms might appear late. Malignant soft tissue tumors occur twice as often as primary bone sarcomas. Approximately 45% of sarcomas occur in the lower extremities, 15% in the upper extremities, 10% in the head-and-neck region, 15% in the retroperitoneum, and the remaining 15% in the abdominal and chest wall. The soft tissue sarcoma can be treated with surgery and if the tumor is unresectable then radiotherapy or chemotherapy can be used.

CASE 96

Abdominal Wall Hernia

CASE

A 55-year-old male with history of painless swelling over left lateral aspect of abdomen in lumbar region since 20 years was referred to the Department of Radiology for CT scan abdomen and pelvis. Six month back he suffered injury from bull's horn on the site of swelling. After that incident the swelling has gradually increased and attained the present size. No history of surgical intervention at the local site.

Radiological Findings on CT Examination

Patient's photograph and X-ray abdomen show swelling in left lateral aspect of abdomen (Figs 1A and B). CT images (Figs 1C and D) show a defect in anterolateral aspect of abdominal wall in left lumbar region with elevation of the external oblique muscle. Omental fat is seen herniating through this defect. No bowel loops or organs are seen to be herniating.

Comments and Explanation

Abdominal wall hernia is protrusion of abdominal structures through the abdominal wall containing (1) an opening in the abdominal wall, and (2) a hernia sac consisting of abdominal contents enclosed by peritoneum. Abdominal wall hernias are a frequent imaging finding in the abdomen. Lumbar hernias occur through defects in the lumbar muscles or the posterior fascia, below the 12th rib and above the iliac crest. They usually occur after surgery or trauma. Diffuse lumbar hernias may also occur, usually after flank incisions in kidney surgery, and may contain bowel loops, retroperitoneal fat, kidneys, or other viscera. Although most abdominal wall hernias are asymptomatic, they may develop acute complications that necessitate emergent surgery. Most cases of bowel obstruction secondary to abdominal wall hernia occur after incarceration and strangulation. CT findings include dilated bowel proximal to the hernia and normal or reduced caliber, or collapsed bowel distal to the obstruction. Strangulation refers to ischemia caused by a compromised blood supply. Findings in ischemia include wall thickening,

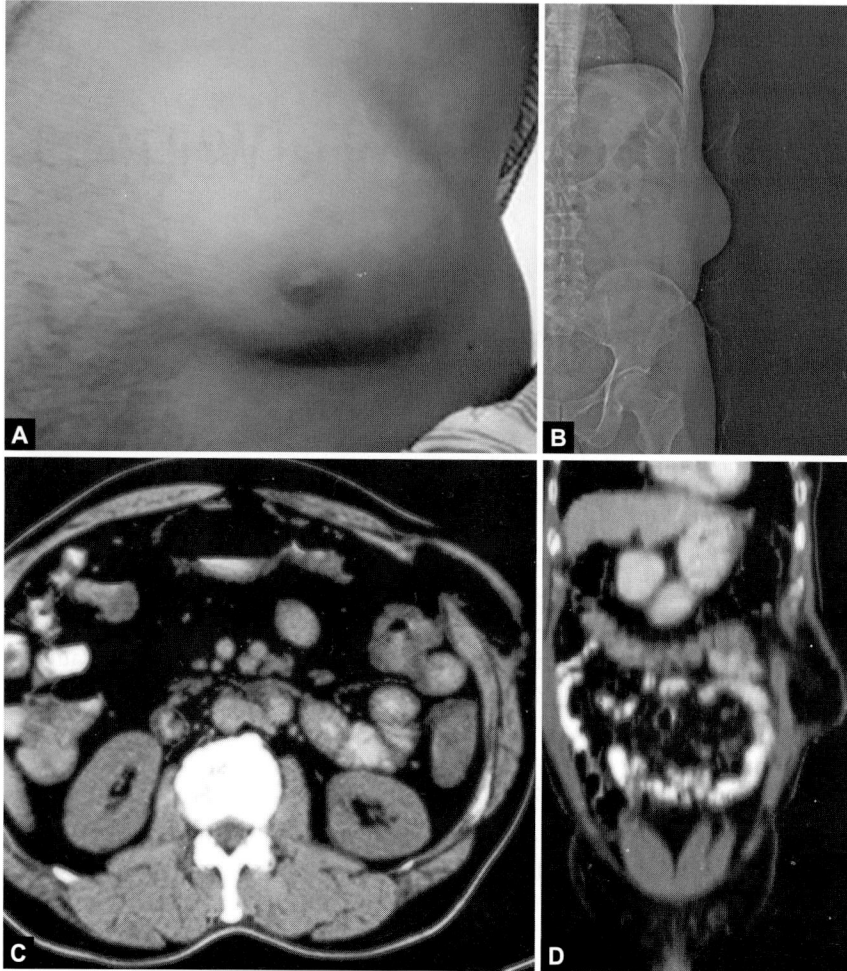

Figs 1A to D

abnormal mural enhancement, mesenteric vessel engorgement, fat obliteration and mesenteric haziness.

Opinion

Abdominal wall hernia.

Clinical Discussion

Types of abdominal wall hernias include inguinal hernia, femoral hernia, ventral hernia, lumbar hernia and incisional hernia. Most common complications of abdominal wall hernias are bowel obstruction secondary to the hernia, incarceration, and strangulation. These complications can often be detected at clinical evaluation. Presenting symptoms may include abdominal pain, vomiting, and distention. Physical examination may reveal a firm, tender abdominal wall mass. Several different surgical procedures are used to repair abdominal wall hernias, ranging from open or laparoscopic suture repair to the use of mesh. To date, tension-free mesh repair has been accepted as the standard surgical technique for the majority of abdominal wall hernias, regardless of defect size and is most commonly used.

SECTION 23

Miscellaneous

97. Inguinal Hernia
98. Omental Infarction
99. Primitive Neuroectodermal Tumor
100. Fetus-in-Fetu
101. Lymphangioma

CASE 97

Inguinal Hernia

CASE

A 50-year-old male with inguinal swelling was subjected to CT abdomen and pelvis.

Radiological Findings on CT Examination

CT scan abdomen shows a large inguinal hernia on right side. Bowel is seen herniating in right scrotal sac (Figs 1A to C). Small inguinal hernia seen on left side (Fig. 1B).

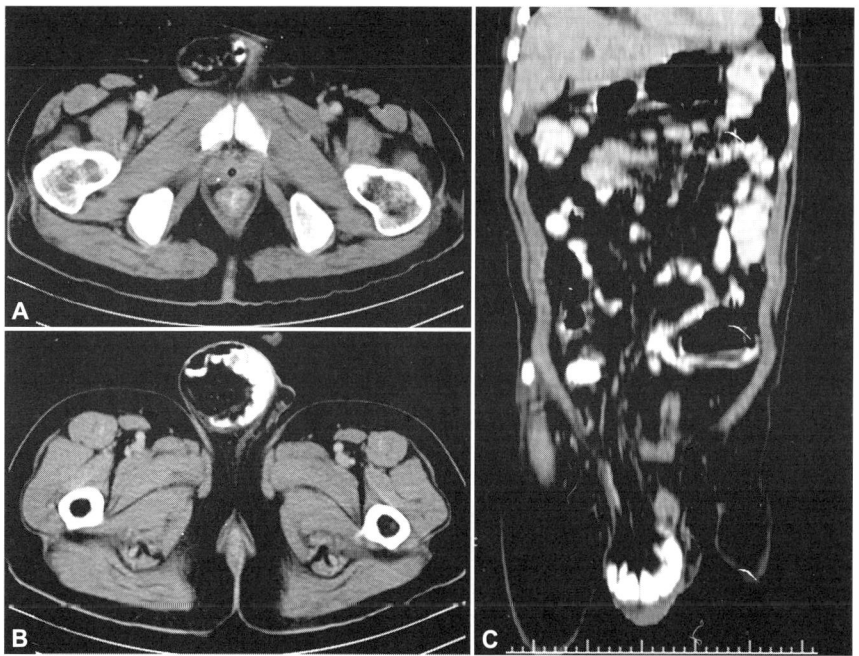

Figs 1A to C

Comments and Explanation

Inguinal hernia is the most common type of hernia and most often acquired. Most commonly occur in males. There are two types of inguinal hernia, direct and indirect. Plain X-ray abdomen shows bowel loop below inguinal ligament. On Sonography and CT examination bowel loops and omentum are seen in inguinal canal. Direct inguinal hernias exit medial and anterior to the course of the inferior epigastric vessels, then are directed inferior to the inferior epigastric vessels as the hernia sac protrudes. They represent a bulge in the anterior abdominal wall lateral to the rectus muscle. The lateral crescent sign on CT represents the laterally displaced and compressed inguinal canal, including its fat and contents. This sign may be less useful in cases of extremely large hernias, which may compress the inguinal canal to such an extent that it may not be readily detectable at CT. Spermatic cord lipomas should not be confused with fat-containing hernias or the lateral crescent sign, as lipomas are typically located lateral or inferior to the spermatic cord and cause no compression of its contents, whereas inguinal hernias protrude anteromedial to the cord. Indirect inguinal hernias are the most common and are caused by the protrusion of peritoneal content through a patent internal inguinal ring, lateral to the inferior epigastric vessels. In men, the hernia can extend along the spermatic cord into the scrotum while in women; the hernia may follow the course of the round ligament into the labia majora. The peritoneal sac containing bowel loops protrudes through the inguinal canal and emerges at the external inguinal ring. Retroperitoneal organs such as the urinary bladder, distal ureters or colon may be incorporated into the hernia.

Opinion

Bilateral inguinal hernia.

Clinical Discussion

Indirect inguinal hernia is commoner and herniates lateral to the inferior epigastric artery, anterior to the spermatic cord in males and follows the round ligament in females. Direct inguinal hernia is less common and herniates medial to the inferior epigastric artery, through a defect in the Hesselbech's triangle. The first sign of an inguinal hernia is a small bulge on one or both sides of the groin, the area just above the groin crease between the lower abdomen and the thigh. The bulge may increase in size over time and usually disappears when lying down. Other signs and symptoms are discomfort or pain in the groin when straining, lifting, coughing, or exercising and improves with rest. Indirect and direct inguinal hernias may slide in and out of the abdomen into the inguinal canal. An incarcerated hernia happens when part of the fat or small intestine from inside the abdomen becomes stuck in the groin or scrotum and cannot go back into the abdomen. When an incarcerated hernia is not treated, the blood supply to the small intestine may become obstructed, causing "strangulation" of the small intestine. This lack of blood supply is an emergency situation and can cause the section of the intestine to die. Open surgery and laparoscopy are treatment options. Inguinal hernias may contain any organ or tissue found in the lower abdomen. These may include but are not limited to fat, small or large bowel, a portion of the bowel wall (Richter hernia), omentum, incarcerated appendix (Amyand hernia), bladder, Meckel's diverticulum (Littré hernia), and gonads. Complications of hernia include intestinal obstruction, incarceration, volvulus, perforation, appendicitis or diverticulitis, and tumors that may be found incidentally in the hernia.

CASE 98

Omental Infarction

CASE

A 60-year-old female with history of pain in abdomen, nausea and vomiting was referred to the department of radiology for CT abdomen and pelvis.

Radiological Findings on CT Examination

Plain and contrast CT abdomen and pelvis shows non enhancing oval essentially fat density omental lesion in the paraumblical region lying posterior to left rectus abdominis muscle measuring 5.6 × 3 cm. There is fat stranding in adjacent surrounding (Figs 1A to D).

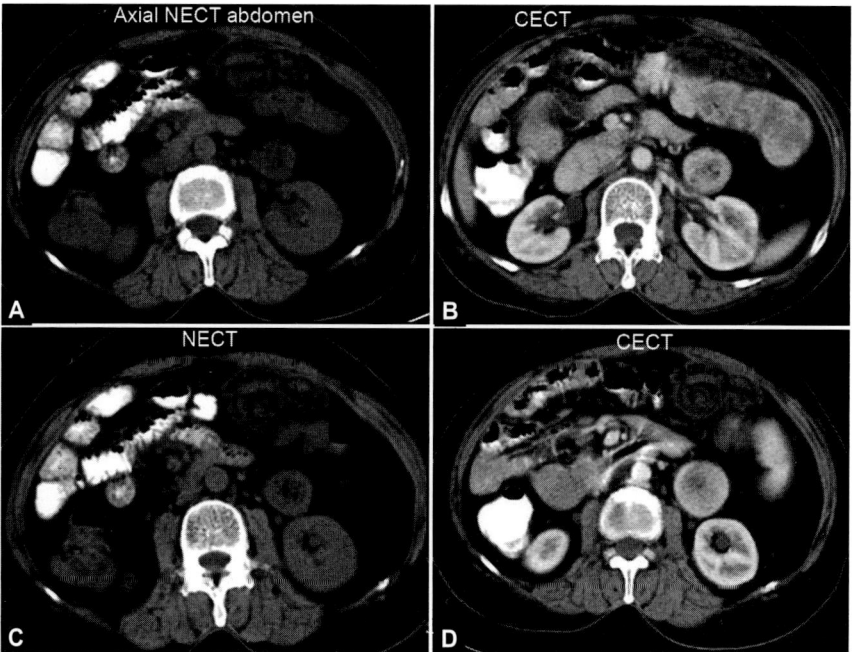

Figs 1A to D

Comments and Explanation

Omental infarction is a rare cause of acute abdomen. Abdominal ultrasound shows focal area of increased echogenicity with fat stranding. CT findings are a solitary large nonenhancing omental mass with heterogeneous attenuation, which is most often located in the right lower quadrant, deep to the rectus abdominis muscle and either anterior to the transverse colon or anteromedial to the ascending colon. Although omental infarction may have a CT appearance that resembles that of acute epiploic appendagitis (Epiploic appendagitis is an uncommon cause of abdominal pain, it is benign, nonsurgical, self-limiting inflammatory process of the epiploic appendices), it lacks the hyperattenuating ring that is seen in epiploic appendagitis. In addition, whereas the central focal lesion in acute epiploic appendagitis is most often less than 5 cm long and is located adjacent to the sigmoid colon, the lesion in omental infarction is larger and most commonly is located next to the cecum or the ascending colon.

Opinion

Omental infarction.

Clinical Discussion

Clinical features are often nonspecific, and the presumptive diagnosis in children is most often appendicitis. Torsion of the omentum, may be primary or secondary. In primary torsion, a mobile segment of omentum rotates around a proximal fixed point in the absence of any associated intra-abdominal pathology. Factors that predispose a patient to torsion include anatomical variations of the omentum itself, e.g. accessory omentum, and narrowed omentum pedicle. Precipitating factors are those causing displacement of the omentum, including trauma, violent exercise, and hyperperistalsis with resultant increased passive movement of the omentum. The omentum twists around a pivotal point, usually in a clockwise direction, venous return is compromised, and the distal omentum becomes congested and edematous. As the torsion progresses arterial occlusion leads to acute hemorragic infarction and eventually necrosis of omentum occurs.

CASE 99

Primitive Neuroectodermal Tumor

CASE

A 32-year-old female presented to the department of radiology with palpable mass in abdomen and pain.

Radiological Findings on CT Examination

CT pelvis (Figs 1A and B) reveal a large heterogeneously enhancing soft tissue density lesion involving the right iliopsoas muscle. A round calcified focus is seen within it. No evidence of fat density within this lesion. The diagnosis of primitive neuroectodermal tumor (PNET) was confirmed on histopathology.

Comments and Explanation

Primitive neuroectodermal tumor (PNET) is rare, highly malignant small-cell neoplasm that most often arises from the chest wall or paravertebral region. Retroperitoneal PNETs tend to be large and aggressive. The imaging characteristic of peripheral PNETs is nonspecific. However, they should be considered in the differential diagnosis for a large, aggressive retroperitoneal mass. Most of them show heterogeneous enhancement with areas of necrosis.

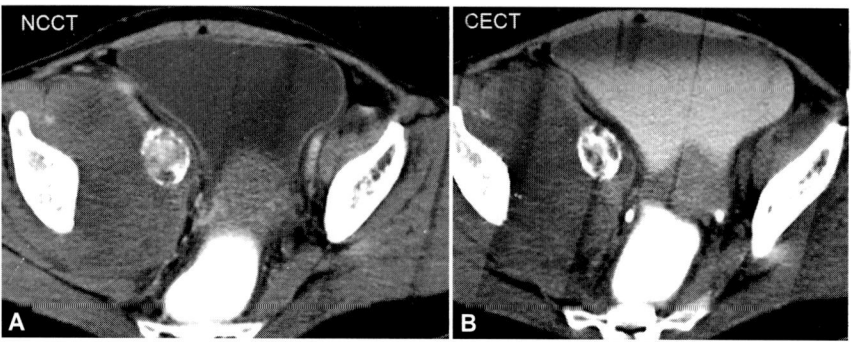

Figs 1A and B

Opinion

Primitive neuroectodermal tumor (PNET).

Clinical Discussion

PNET is a malignant neural crest tumor. It usually occurs in children and young adults under 25 years of age. The Askin tumor, a PNET of the chest wall, is seen mostly among children and adolescents. It is closely related to Ewing's sarcoma of the same location, both tumors showing the same chromosomal translocation. Pain and deformity of the chest wall are the cardinal clinical signs of the tumor. Askin tumors show a female predilection, with typical presentation being in the second decade.

PNET gets its name because the majority of the cells in the tumor are derived from neuroectoderm; it is classified into two types, based on location in the body: peripheral PNET and CNS PNET. The peripheral PNET is now thought to be virtually identical to Ewing sarcoma. PNETs of the CNS generally refer to supratentorial PNETs.

CASE 100

Fetus-in-Fetu

CASE

A 5-year-old male presented with palpable mass in abdomen and was referred to the department of radiology for CT scan abdomen and pelvis.

Radiological Findings on CT Examination

X-ray abdomen reveal a large well demarcated mass occupying a large central part of upper abdomen with few dense linear structures (Fig. 1A) CT abdomen reveal a large heterogeneous density mass lesion in the peritoneal cavity displacing the normal structures. The mass has solid, cystic, fatty and osseous components. Few well formed tubular bones and joints are seen (Figs 1B and C), the fat plane between the lesion and adjacent abdominal structures is well maintained. Complete surgical excision of the lesion (Fig. 1D) was performed and the diagnosis was confirmed on histopathology.

Comments and Explanation

Fetus-in-fetu is an extremely rare abnormality that occurs secondary to abnormal embryogenesis in a monochorionic diamniotic pregnancy where a nonviable fetus becomes enclosed within a normally developing fetus. Most occur in the abdomen/retroperitoneal cavity, CT typically shows an abdominal mass with some components favoring fetal parts within the abdomen of another neonate.

Opinion

Fetus-in-fetu.

Clinical Discussion

Imaging plays an important role to correctly diagnose evaluates the case in a prospective manner. The diagnosis of fetus in fetu can be made with abdominal conventional radiographs, by identifying a vertebral column and/or specific bony

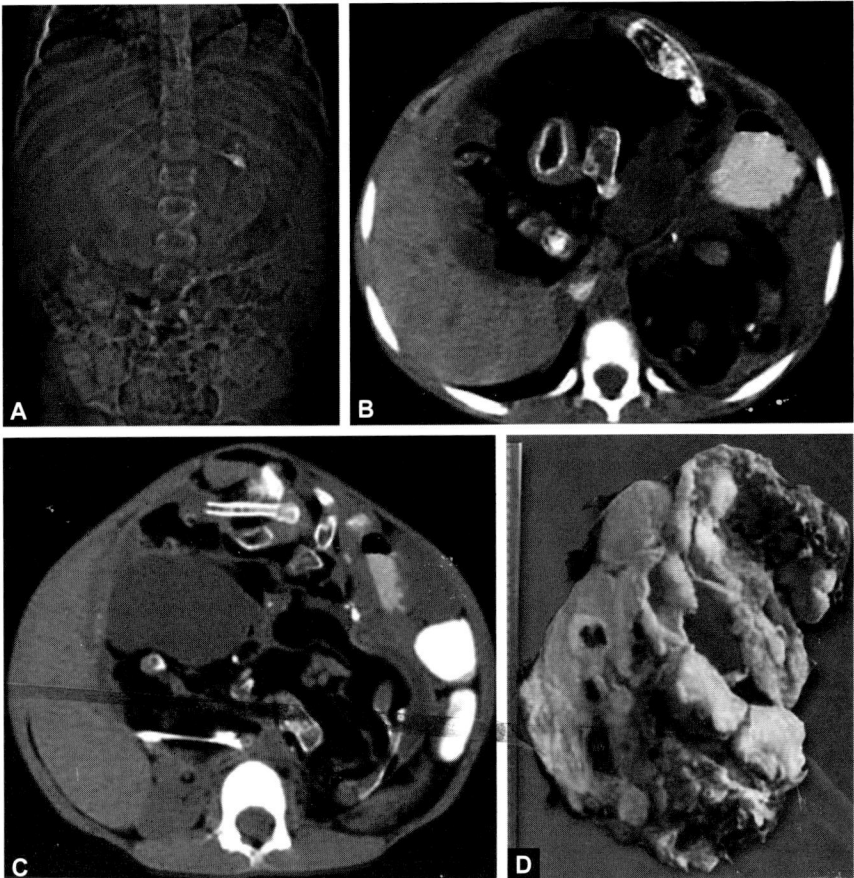

Figs 1A to D *(For color version D, see plate 4)*

structures. The CT findings are those of a mass that consisted of a round or tubular collection of fat that surrounded a central bony structure. The identification of vertebrae or long bones is essential for establishing this diagnosis prospectively. This entity is distinguished from an intrabdominal teratoma by its embryological origin, its unusual location in the retroperitoneal space, its invariable benignity, and by the presence of vertebral organization with limb buds and well-developed organ systems. The most important feature that has been used to distinguish between fetus-in-fetu and teratoma is the presence of a vertebral column. Identification of the vertebral column indicates that fetal development of the included twin must have advanced at least to the primitive streak stage to develop a notochord, which is the precursor of the vertebral column.

CASE 101

Lymphangioma

CASE

A young 18-year-old male patient complaining of pain in left iliac region since one year was referred to radiology department for CT scan abdomen.

Radiological Findings on CT Scan

CT abdomen and pelvis (Figs 1A to D) show ill defined fluid density lesion with imperceptible wall in the retroperitoneum surrounding the aorta and IVC.

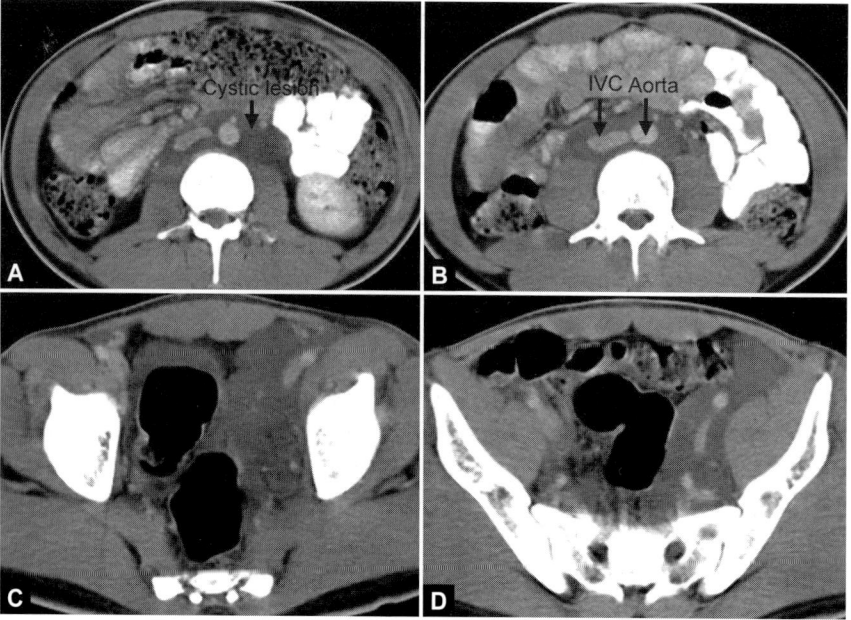

Figs 1A to D

It extends along the left iliac vessels into the left half of pelvis. No evidence of enhancement is seen in this lesion. Surrounding fat planes are preserved. This lesion represents lymphangioma.

Comments and Explanation

Lymphangiomas are benign lesions of vascular origin that show lymphatic differentiation. They occur in many anatomic locations and may have a pediatric or adult clinical presentation. After birth, they can become markedly dilated as a result of both the collection of fluid and the budding of pre-existing spaces. They may form unilocular or multilocular cystic masses and can encroach on vital structures. Sonographically, lymphangiomas are most often multilocular cystic masses that are anechoic or contain echogenic debris. At CT, cystic lymphangioma typically appears as a large, thin-walled, multiseptate cystic mass. Its attenuation values varies from that of fluid to that of fat. If hemorrhage occurs, the intracystic attenuation values may simulate a solid tumor mass or abscess. An elongated shape and crossing from one retroperitoneal compartment to an adjacent one are characteristic of the mass. Rarely, cystic lymphangiomas may have wall calcification. Signal pattern of lymphangiomas on MRI resembles that of fluid: low signal intensity on T1W images and high signal intensity on T2W images. The presence of hemorrhage or infection in the lesion may alter the MRI signal pattern to give a more solid appearance.

Opinion

Lymphangioma.

Clinical Discussion

Lymphangiomas are benign congenital abnormalities of the lymphatic system. They are thought to arise from sequestrations of embryonic lymph sacs; these sacs are found in the neck and retroperitoneum. 75% of lymphangiomas occur in the neck. Lymphangiomatosis is a rare disease with multifocal lymphatic proliferation that typically presents during childhood and involves multiple parenchyma organs including the lung, liver, spleen, bone, and skin. Because lymphangiomas present across a wide age range of patient ages and occur in many sites, they are associated with a broad spectrum of clinical and radiologic manifestations. The acute presentation of lymphangiomas can cause abdominal pain, tenderness, distension, fever, leukocytosis, peritonitis, dysuria, and guarding. The abnormal ducts vary in size from microscopic to several centimeters and there is a variable component of fibrous adventitia. The large cystic lesions are also known as cystic hygromas. Surgical excision is the treatment of choice. The long-term prognosis is excellent if complete excision has been achieved.

Index

A

Abdomen 11, 100, 103, 178, 199
  acute 301
    pain in 27, 29, 173
  distension of 70
  severe pain in 45
Abdominal wall hernias, types of 292
Abscess 167
  appendicular 63, 64
  formation 63
  hepatic 97, 98
  pyogenic 97
  splenic 166, 167
Acalculous cholecystitis 131, 132, 134
Adenocarcinoma 35, 41, 54, 81, 283
  duodenal 42
  ileal 54
  mucinous 285
Adenoma 54
  adrenal 189
  hepatic 108, 109
Adenopathy, peripheral 48
Adrenocorticotropic hormone 190
Adult polycystic kidney disease 204
Aganglionosis, intestinal 264
Agenesis, renal 200, 264
Alcohol abuse 148
American Association for Surgery of Trauma 95, 219, 220
American Joint Committee on Cancer 228
Ampulla of Vater 155
Androgen 254
Anemia 75
Angiodysplasia 52
Angiomyolipoma 110, 111
  hepatic 110, 111
  renal 221, 222
Antiphospholipid syndrome 93
Aorta 171
  abdominal 174, 177-179, 182, 183
Aortic aneurysm, abdominal 179
Aortic dissection 204
Aortic thrombus 182
  infrarenal 183
Aplasia
  renal 199
  uterovaginal 200
Appendicitis 61, 62
Appendix 13, 57
Apple core sign 54
Arteries
  abdominal 177
  mesenteric 177
  renal 14
  stenosis, renal 176
Ascaris lumbricoides 139
Askin tumors 303
Aspergillosis 93
Autoimmune disease 132
Autoimmune disorders 56
Autosomal dominant polycystic kidney disease 204

B

Balthazar score 148
Beckwith-Wiedemann syndrome 119
Behçet's disease 93
Berry's aneurysm, cerebral 204
Bicornuate uterus 264
Biliary cirrhosis 130, 139
Biliary injury 96
Black pigment stones 139
Bladder 299
  diverticulum 233
Blunt abdominal trauma 219
Blunt injury 250
Bowel injuries 163
Broad ligament 15
  fibroid 261
Brood capsules 101
Budd-Chiari syndrome 91, 92, 126

C

Calculus cholecystitis 133, 134
Cancer
  cervical 270, 277
  colorectal 78
  esophageal 22
  rectal 82
Carcinoma
  cervix 270, 271
  colorectal 78
  duodenum 41
  endometrial 267, 268
  esophageal 21, 22

gallbladder 142, 143
gastric 36
hepatocellular 110, 112, 113, 117, 126
ileal 53
penile 257, 258
periampullary 155
prostate 243, 244
rectal 82
rectum 81
sigmoid 77
    colon 78
stomach 35, 36
urinary bladder 237, 239
vulval 276, 277
Cardiovascular disorders 132
Caroli disease 121
Cecum 57
Celiac trunk 177
Cell carcinoma, renal 181, 226, 227
Cholangiocarcinoma 120, 121, 123, 124
    extrahepatic 123, 124
    intrahepatic 120, 121
Cholangitis 122, 130, 139
    primary sclerosing 121, 139
Cholecystitis 134, 141
    acute 134
    calcifying 141
    emphysematous 136, 137, 141
Cholecystocholedochal fistula 141
Cholecystopathia chronica calcarea 141
Choledochal cyst 129, 130
Choledocholithiasis 130, 138, 139
Cholelithiasis 130, 140, 141
Cloacal exstrophy 254
Clonorchis sinensis 139
Cluster sign 98
Colon 65
Common iliac artery, bilateral 183
Computed tomography scan 33, 92, 100, 112
    abdomen 1, 23, 27, 33, 35, 47, 51, 55, 57, 61, 63, 67, 74, 77, 81, 89, 97, 91, 106, 110, 115, 118, 129, 147, 149, 201, 205, 263
    chest 27
    pelvis 1, 61, 63, 74, 97, 106, 115, 118
    renal angiography 176
    thorax 23
Constipation, chronic 53
Contrast enhanced computed tomography scan 70, 94, 201, 265
    abdomen 51, 67, 91, 142, 149, 272
    pelvis 272
Couinaud classification of liver 1
Crescent sign 179, 183
Crohn's disease 42, 46, 75
Cyst 204
    multiple 203
    rupture 204
    simple hepatic 89, 90

Cystitis 235, 236
    acute 236
    cystica 236
    glandularis 236
Cysto-biliary fistulas 102
Cystolithiasis 130
Cystourethrogram, micturating 234

D

Daughter vesicles 101
Diabetes
    gestational 254
    mellitus 132
Diaphragm 25
    eventration of 28, 29
Diarrhea 68
Distension, abdominal 41
Diverticulitis 73
    sigmoid 72, 73
Diverticulosis, colonic 204
Dolichoectasia, intracranial 204
Doughnut sign 68
Duodenum 57
Dysphagia 21, 23

E

Emphysema, surgical 163
End stage renal failure 204
Endometrium, high grade carcinoma of 267
Escherichia coli 215, 236
Esophageal carcinoma, staging of 22
Esophagus, leiomyomatosis of 23
Ewing's sarcoma 303
Extracorporeal shock wave lithotripsy 209

F

Fallopian tubes 15
Familial adenomatous polyposis 42, 119
Fatigue 48
Fecal occult blood test 82
Fetal alcohol syndrome 119
Fever 75
Fistula
    pancreatic 155
    ureterovaginal 274
Flank pain, severe 209
Fluoro-2-deoxy-D-glucose 251
Focal fatty liver 87
Foramen of Winslow 14

G

Galactosemia syndrome 92
Gallbladder 5
    carcinoma 139, 143, 144
    phrygian cap 5

polyp 139
porcelain 139-141, 144
wall, calcification of 141
Gallstone 148
ileus 141
Gardner's syndrome 42, 54, 119
Gastroesophageal junction 20, 21
Gastrointestinal stromal tumor 33, 34, 49, 50
Gastrointestinal system 9
Gastrointestinal tract 33
Genitourinary malformations 119
Germ cell tumor 252
Gerota's fascia 147, 228
Glycogen storage disease 119

H

Hayfork sign 68
Helicobacter pylori infection 35
Hemangioma 103, 104, 126
hepatic 103
Hematemesis, complaints of 35
Hematoma 94-96
parenchymal 163
subcapsular hepatic 163
Hematosalpinx 264
Hematuria 220
Hemoglobinuria, paroxysmal nocturnal 93
Hemoperitoneum 94, 163, 164
Hemorrhage 118, 156, 204
Hepatectomy, partial 114
Hepatic cyst, benign developmental 90
Hepatitis B 114
Hepatitis C 114
Hepatoblastoma 118, 119
Hiatus hernia 19, 20
Hounsfield units 190
Human papillomavirus infection 277
Hutch diverticulum 233
Hydatid cyst 100, 101
hepatic 100, 101
Hydatid disease, hepatic 101
Hydrocele 247
bilateral 247, 248
Hydrometrocolpos 263, 264
Hydronephrosis 274
proximal 206
Hyperplasia
fibronodular 112
focal nodular 106, 107, 115, 126
lymphoid 62
Hypertension, portal 130, 186

I

Inguinal hernia 297, 298
bilateral 298
indirect 298

Inguinal lymphadenectomy 258
Intussusception, colocolic 68
Ischemia 61

J

Jejunum 57
angiodysplasia of 51, 52

K

Kidney
dysplastic 201
failure 119
ureters, and bladder 212, 232
Klebsiella pneumoniae 215
Krukenberg tumor 35

L

Labia majora 277
Labia minora 277
Laceration
renal 219, 220
splenic 163
Leukemia 116
Ligament of Treitz 9
Littré hernia 299
Liver 1
biopsy 92
focal fatty infiltration of 87, 88
function tests 117
laceration 94
parenchyma, adjacent 143
segments, anatomy of 1
Lump, abdominal 63
Lung carcinoma, primary 194
Lymph node
metastasis 273
prepyloric 35
Lymphadenopathy
mediastinal 48
regional 48
Lymphangioma 306, 307
Lymphoid tissue 76
Lymphoma 35, 47
ileocecal 47
small bowel 47

M

Mackenrodt's ligament 15
Mayer-Rokitansky-Küster-Hauser syndrome 264
McBurney's point 62
McKusick-Kaufman syndrome 264
Meckel's diverticulum 299
Mesenteric artery thrombosis, acute 175
Metastases
adrenal 194

hepatic 41, 115, 116, 244
nodal 239
Midgut volvulus 57
Mirizzi syndrome 141
Müllerian duct anomalies 200, 264
Multicystic dysplastic kidney 202
Multiple endocrine neoplasia 193
Murphy's sign 134
Myometrium 14
Myxedemic ileus, acute 71

N

Necrosis 61
    pancreatic 154
Neoplastic polyps 78
Nephroblastoma 224
Neurofibromatosis 193
Non-Hodgkin's lymphoma 47
    ileocecal 47
Non-steroidal anti-inflammatory drugs 209
Noonan syndrome 254
North American National Wilms' Tumor Study Group 224

O

Obstruction, small bowel 45, 46
Ogilive's syndrome 71
Omental infarction 300, 301
Organ of Zuckerkandl 193
Organs
    abdominal 94
    injury, abdominal 163
Ovarian neoplasms 284
Ovarian tumor 283, 285
    epithelial 284
Ovarian vein thrombosis 281, 282
    bilateral 282

P

Pain
    abdominal 41, 82, 189
    acute 204
    hypochondriac 136
    intermittent abdominal 202
Pancreas 8, 145
    enlargement of 148
Pancreatitis 139, 148, 156
    acute 147, 148, 154
    necrotizing 153, 154
    severe acute 154
Papillary mucinous tumors, intraductal 151
Parasites 62
Pelvic calculus, renal 208
Pelvis 178

female 13
male 15
Pelviureteric junction 206, 207
    obstruction 205, 207
Peutz-Jhegers syndrome 54
Peyer's patches 76
Pheochromocytoma 192, 193
    adrenal 193
Pneumatosis intestinalis 55, 56
Pneumoperitoneum 73
Polycystic kidney 203
    bilateral 203
    disease 204
Portal vein thrombosis 184-186
Positron emission tomography 120, 251
Post-Whipple's surgery 155
Potter syndrome 200
Pouch of Douglas 15
Prader-Willi syndrome 254
Prostate 243
    cancer 244
    specific antigen tests 244
Prune-Belly syndrome 254
Pseudoaneurysm 96, 148
Pseudocyst 148-150, 152
    pancreatic 149, 151
Pyelography, intravenous 232
Pyelonephritis, emphysematous 215, 218
Pyometra 265, 266
    causes of 266

R

Renal pelvic calculus 209
Reye's syndrome 92
Rib fracture 163
Richter hernia 299
Roux-en-Y hepaticojejunostomy 130

S

Sarcoma 35
    abdominal 290
Scleroderma 56
Scoliosis 171
Seminoma 251
Shock, hemorrhagic 222
Small bowel wall, multiple segments of 55
Small intestine, primary neoplasms of 54
Sphincter of Oddi 8, 130
Spleen 8, 164
    abscess of 167
Splenic vein, thrombosis of 184
Squamous cell carcinoma 22, 239, 257, 272, 276
Staghorn calculi 210, 211
    bilateral 210
Stomach 21, 31
Sturge-Weber syndrome 193

Superior mesenteric artery 57, 58, 171
    syndrome 171, 173, 175
Superior mesenteric vein 57
    thrombosis of 184

T

Testes, undescended 253, 254
Testicular seminoma 251
Thrombosis 174
Todani classification system 130
Trauma
    hepatic 94
    renal 219
    splenic 163
    testicular 249
Tuberculosis
    abdominal 75
    gastrointestinal 75
    pulmonary 75
Tuberous sclerosis 193
Tumors 62
    adrenal 193
    periampullary 157
    small bowel 54

U

Ulcerative colitis 121
Ultrasonography, transrectal 244
Upper gastrointestinal system 9
Ureteric calculus 212
Urinary bladder diverticulum 233
Urinary tract infection, recurrent 202, 204, 234

Urogenital sinus 264
Urogram, intravenous 206
Uropathy, obstructive 208
Uterine didelphys 264
Uterosacral ligament 15
Uterovesicle pouch 15

V

Vaginal bleeding 270
Vaginal carcinoma 272, 273
Vaginal discharge 270
Vein thrombosis, renal 217, 218
Vena cava
    inferior 180
    superior 180
Vesical calculus 231, 232
Vesicoureteric reflux 234
Vesicoureteric junction calculi, bilateral 213
Vomiting 29
von Hippel-Lindau disease 193
von Meyenburg complex 90
Vulvar cancer, primary 276

W

Whipple's surgery 155
Whirlpool' appearance 57
Wilms' tumor 116, 119, 181, 223, 224, 225

Z

Zoonosis, parasitic 101